BODY BY FERRARI

HOW TO GET THE BEST RESULTS FROM YOUR BODY CONTOURING PROCEDURES

Victor S. Ferrari, MD, FACS

Acknowledgements

I first want to thank my Lord and Savior, Jesus Christ for dying on a cross to forgive me of my sins. Therefore, I can have a relationship with the Living God now and forevermore in Heaven. I also want to thank my wife and children for making my life joyful and encouraging me every day to live each day to the fullest.

Also, I want to thank the late Dr. Ralph Millard, Jr. He was my mentor and world-renowned plastic surgeon who taught me to know what is considered beautiful and then be able to change the physical aspects of someone's face or body to make them more beautiful.

Contents

Why You Should Read This Book

If you've been considering altering a facial or body feature to improve your appearance, you are not alone. Throughout recorded history, humans have had procedures described to improve their looks. Every year, millions of Americans undergo cosmetic procedures to enhance their looks, boost their self-esteem, or just feel more confident in social settings. Multiple studies have clearly shown that people that are more attractive have higher income, more confidence, higher employment rates, and greater ease in social settings. Attractive people also have an easier time getting others to help them, have an easier time getting hired for jobs, and are typically seen as more intelligent and competent. We may not like the results of these studies, but the emotional, social, physical, and economic benefits of being more beautiful can't be denied.

I personally have seen over 40,000 patients in my career and have written this book to help people through this important life-changing process. With proper education and understanding, comes the ability to make wise decisions regarding your health and pursuit of beauty. Those who are poorly informed run a much higher risk of making a bad choice of procedure or provider, either of which could lead to making you less attractive. Unfortunately, I have had to correct hundreds of "botched" surgeries over the years from those who made such errors in judgment at the hands of unqualified or unscrupulous physicians. My hope is that if even one person is saved from doctor-induced deformity by reading this book, it will all be worth it.

After performing plastic surgery for over 20 years, I am still amazed at how many of my patients come to me for consultation and have been given very little information at other offices with respect to the surgical procedure they are considering. Some doctors load up their schedules with so many patients, they simply don't have time to give full disclosure on what's involved when having surgery. In order for you to make wise, informed decisions about your health, you need to be given enough information to be able to weigh the pros and cons of every procedure you choose (or refuse) to undergo. Certainly you can do some basic research on your own such as on the Internet, but details are often scanty. So, if you've been considering having a cosmetic procedure, I invite you to read this book (or at least the sections that are pertinent to your area of interest) and educate yourself as much as possible before you decide on which procedure is best for you and which physician you will allow to change your appearance.

Regardless of whether or not you come to my office for your care, this book can help you understand what's involved, red flags to avoid, and discerning questions you should be asking before making your final decision. It will help you to navigate through the "cosmetic waters" so you will have a thorough understanding of what's involved in your decision, what to expect from your desired procedure, realistic outcomes, and most importantly, choosing the right physician. By understanding what's involved, you will be empowered to avoid making serious mistakes. I have seen these mistakes hundreds of times by patients that were poorly informed about their procedure or chose a doctor that was not properly qualified for the procedure they had in mind. In addition, by choosing the right procedure and the right practitioner, you may greatly decrease your chances of having to undergo a painful and quite possibly expensive secondary corrective surgery.

A classic tragic example occurred when I was in my second year of private practice. A thirty-two year old female came to my office six days after having undergone a breast augmentation in another country. She had traveled there because she was saving approximately $1,500. She was feverish and felt light-headed. A physical exam revealed pain, redness, and swelling of both breasts. She was taken immediately to surgery. As soon as I made the first incision into her right breast, yellow-green foul-smelling pus came pouring out. The left side had a similar situation. After removing both implants, she spent 3 days in the hospital on IV antibiotics.

Four months later, she underwent breast augmentation again, but this time with me. Even though she had saved $1,500 by going to another country, her final bill, after the breast implant removal, hospitalization, and re-augmentation was over $22,000, and that does not even include her lost wages for time off work. If she had made a properly informed and educated decision, she would not have gone overseas to have her surgery. She would have gladly spent the extra money the first time she had her surgery if she had a clear understanding of all the issues involved. The take-home message is that getting things done right the first time is your most cost-effective and best chance of getting the result you want. So, follow the guidelines in this book to maximize your chance of getting the look you desire in the most cost-effective way with the easiest and shortest recovery.

Another reason to read this book is to increase your comfort level. Educated patients are more realistic and have greater comfort in understanding the process and recovery associated with each procedure they choose. Therefore, they can more accurately make scheduling plans in terms of time off work, social events, vacations, etc.

In addition, reading this book will help you be a more discerning "shopper". In other words, not only will you have a better understanding of the procedures, you will also be able to determine if your doctor is properly suited to perform your procedure. You need to realize that as insurance reimbursement to doctors continues to decline, more and more physicians will scramble to get the minimal amount of training in order to do cosmetic procedures. They will have slick marketing and call themselves "board-certified," but you need to be able to evaluate what that really means. I hope to be able to educate you as to who has appropriate credentials and therefore is worthy of your trust and who is not. Making the wrong choice of a provider could lead to irreversible disfigurement so please take the time to do your "homework" before you decide.

I have included a number of before-and-after comparisons in this book. A number of additional representative comparisons of some of my patients can be seen in a photo gallery at http://www.Natural-LookingResults.com/Photo-Gallery.

CHAPTER 1

What Is Beauty and Why Does it Matter?

The human race has been in search for beauty for thousands of years. When I began researching the material for this book, I realized that ever since people have been living together in community settings, there was evidence that they tried to make themselves more beautiful in the eyes of others. Sometimes, it involved just certain clothing or headdressing. Other times, it involved painting, tattooing, scarring, mutilation, tanning, skin bleaching, tooth whitening, implanting gems or gold into teeth, or plastic surgery. So, how exactly do we define beauty? *Beauty* has proven to be an elusive term, which cannot transcend time or cultural boundaries. In other words, beauty, like fashion, is typically defined by our own particular culture and definitely changes over time. Religious preferences can also dictate what we deem as attractive. For example, the Greeks and Romans saw the naked body as beautiful and commonly displayed it in their art. At a different time, the Victorians saw the naked body as sinful and lustful; therefore, Victorian art always had their subjects fully clothed.

Wikipedia defines it this way: *"Beauty* is a characteristic of a person, animal, place, object, or idea that provides a perceptual experience of pleasure or satisfaction. *Beauty* is studied as part of aesthetics, sociology, social psychology, and culture. An *ideal beauty* is an entity, which is admired, or possesses features widely attributed to beauty in a particular culture, for perfection. The experience of *beauty* often involves an interpretation of some entity as being in balance and harmony with nature, which may lead to feelings of attraction and emotional well-being. Because this can be a subjective experience, it is often said, 'beauty is in the eye of the beholder'."

There is evidence that many of our perceptions of beauty actually begin in early childhood. As we looked at our parent's faces or bodies, we started developing ideas about what is considered beautiful. Over time, our perceptions change depending on external influences, which have caused us pleasure or satisfaction.

Mathematicians have attempted to define beauty according to certain proportions. They have developed the concept of "the golden ratio" also known as "phi." Cosmetic surgeons are not the only ones who use the "golden ratio" to try to enhance beauty. Other professionals, such as architects, landscapers, and car designers also use the "phi" ratio as well. For humans, symmetry has been perceived as beautiful, quite possibly because it subliminally indicates the absence of genetic defects.

Human beauty is not only defined by outward appearance, but by a person's "inner beauty." Inner beauty refers to any combination of characteristics we find attractive such as personality, kindness, unselfishness, intelligence, politeness, grace, integrity, elegance, etc. We can all think of someone who was not physically attractive but their inner beauty made them beautiful in our eyes. In other words, inner beauty can trump outer beauty. Though inner beauty is very important, that is not the focus of this book.

We are all keenly aware that the media greatly influences what we consider physically beautiful. Every week, we typically see hundreds of examples of what is considered "beautiful." As a result, we have developed a keen eye for what we want. For example, women no longer just want thinner arms. They want arms that have a shape like those of Michelle Obama or Jennifer Anniston. It's not just size that matters; shape, skin texture, and color also make a difference in what we perceive as beautiful. As a result, the general population has become more specific, and in many ways more demanding, in terms of what they want to achieve when it comes to aesthetic transformation.

If beauty is such an elusive, ever changing concept, why does it matter? Why are we seeking the "holy grail" of beauty? Why is the pursuit of beauty so important that people will sacrifice time, expense, and physical pain to achieve it? The answer lies in how society perceives beauty. We use beauty to compare one person with another and rightly or wrongly, we make initial quick judgments about that person based on their appearance. We instantly decide if this person is a friend or foe. Culturally, our personal definition of beauty separates "us" from "them."

Our physical appearance and the way we dress also is a powerful form of communication. In an unspoken discourse, we broadcast to the world what we're all about by the way we look. We signal to each other things such as compatibility, nationality, intelligence, femininity or masculinity, occupation, social status, accomplishments, wealth, health, youthfulness, hygiene, fitness, lifestyle, preferences, sexual prowess, and even possibly political affiliation. Our appearance is linked to our personal identity. If you perceive that your appearance and identity are in conflict, then you will be motivated to undergo whatever it takes to get yourself "in sync."

Beauty also has many other benefits in all societies and cultures. More often than not, the world rewards beautiful people. Various studies have shown that those who are considered physically attractive typically have an easier time getting a job, make more money, and are generally tolerated for their personality flaws to a higher degree than their less attractive counterparts. Beautiful people also do better in sales or politics. Fine-looking people are also perceived as being healthier, more intelligent, more competent, more persuasive, more likeable, and more trustworthy. Attractive people also have an easier time finding a mate because good looks signal youth, health, and reproductive fitness. In addition, people are typically more eager to help out an attractive person in need.

So, whether we like it or not, beautiful people have an easier time making it through all aspects of life. They also have advantages and can open doors to opportunities based on their appearance alone. We may not think it's fair, but it's just the way it is. So for these reasons, beauty does matter and the personal pursuit of beauty has its' own rewards.

CHAPTER 2

Are You Considering a Change?

Most people have some physical aspect of their face or body that they wouldn't mind changing. The question is, at what point does that feature bother you enough to motivate you to go out and do something about it? For some, it's as simple as losing weight. For others, there are genetic or traumatic events that have given them an unfavorable appearance. When deciding on a course of action, we typically consider the pros and cons of action vs. inaction. When the pain of doing nothing exceeds the pain of taking action, then a decision to proceed with change follows. Or, conversely, when the expectation of happiness, satisfaction, or pleasure associated with making a change exceeds the dissatisfaction of not making a change, then change will occur. So, in essence, we all make decisions hoping to maximize our pleasure and minimize our pain.

Making a decision to undergo any surgical procedure should be done after careful consideration. The first thing to decide is if you are properly motivated to undergo a cosmetic procedure. In other words, are you doing this to feel better about your appearance or are you trying to satisfy someone else's desires or obtain some ideal image in your mind, which might not ever be attainable? If you feel you are properly motivated psychologically and have realistic expectations, then there are physical issues to consider. The best candidates are healthy, have stable weight, and are non-smokers.

As you consider having a cosmetic procedure performed, it's wise to again pause and consider why you are doing it. If you are motivated by a personal pursuit of happiness and have a clear idea of what you want to accomplish, then the next step is to consider the risks and costs associated with your decision. The degree of risk will, in part, be determined by the provider you select, as will be discussed in this book. If your motivation for a change in physical appearance is that you hope that some other aspect of your life will improve, then you may be terribly disappointed despite an overall favorable aesthetic result. For example, if you are hoping that cosmetic surgery will help salvage your relationship with your "significant other," you may want to reconsider what you are doing. Any relationship that is based mainly on physical attraction may not be worth salvaging. So, be honest with yourself, and ask yourself why you want to make a change.

You should also be aware of a mental disorder called "Body Dysmorphic Disorder" or "BDD." This is a chronic mental illness in which individuals are excessively concerned about a perceived defect in their physical appearance, which is typically considered a minor or imagined flaw. Often, these people develop depression, anxiety, social withdrawal, social isolation, obsessive-compulsive disorders, and even thoughts of suicide. BDD affects about 1% of the population and seems to be fairly equally distributed between males and females. If you think you may have this problem, it's best to seek psychiatric help before ever undergoing a cosmetic procedure.

Be sure you have realistic expectations regarding the procedure you are considering. This is something you definitely need to discuss with your doctor. Be careful not to base your expectations on what you have seen on the Internet or what your friends have told you. There is a lot of bad and outright deceitful information online. For example, you will see examples of liposuction where the "after" photo looks like the patient has lost a lot of weight. The fact is that patient may have lost a lot of weight by their own efforts, after the surgery was performed. But, when you look at the photos, you are led to believe that it was all due to the skill of the surgeon and that is just not the case.

Your age and overall health also need to be taken into account especially when considering surgery. Smoking, diabetes, obesity, sedentary lifestyle, poor nutrition, blood clotting disorders, heart disease, lung disease, or any other medical conditions, all need to be factored in when deciding on surgery. Your primary doctor may need to be consulted to be sure you are healthy enough for surgery.

If you feel that you are properly motivated, have realistic expectations, are sufficiently healthy, and you don't have BDD, then the next question is the timing of your procedure. For example, if you have always wanted a tummy tuck, but still want to have more children, it would be best to wait until your childbearing days are over. Or, if you have a significant social event planned in the near future such as a wedding, you may want to be sure to allow enough time for the healing process to be complete before your big day. There are also seasonal considerations to take into account. For instance, laser skin resurfacing is best done in the fall and winter months so you won't be out in the sun much during the early healing phase. If you're not sure if your timing is right, be sure to ask your plastic surgeon before proceeding.

CHAPTER 3

How to Find a Qualified Plastic Surgeon

In our world of slick Internet and social media marketing, many patients are duped into thinking that someone is a hero, when, in fact, they're something much less. Beautiful websites lure us in and convince us that we're in expert hands. Some are truthful, but some are not. I even had one doctor "borrow" my photos off of my website and post them as his own work. When I confronted him, he said he would tell patients that the photos were examples of what could be possible, but claims he never said they were his own work. Obviously, the fact that he posted them on his website was a way of making patients think that he had done the work himself.

So how do you know if a plastic surgeon is qualified or not? One excellent way is to talk it over with friends to see if they have any insight as to who is good or not. Hair stylists, nurses, aestheticians, or other medical personnel are also good resources of information. Online reviews can also be helpful. If you have the good fortune of being able to talk with a former patient, this too would be extremely valuable.

What about board certification? Almost every doctor will tout that he or she is "board certified." The question you must ask is "what is the name of the board that certified you?" All board certifications are not created equal. And, you do not need to be board certified in plastic surgery to be able to perform plastic surgery. In other words, someone could be a gynecologist who performs plastic surgery procedures and is board certified by the American Board of Obstetrics and Gynecology. Therefore, he can honestly say he is "board certified," but not tell you that it's not in plastic surgery.

If the physician you are considering has a board certification in something that has the word "cosmetic" in it, I would advise you to "beware." Some of these board certifications have been obtained by doctors that have had minimal training to learn how to do some plastic surgery procedure. For example, I once had a patient with a terrible complication from breast augmentation. One implant was about 2 inches higher than the other. When I questioned her as to who did her surgery, she told me her doctor was an expert in breast augmentation with "board certification." When I researched information about her physician, I found out he was an emergency room doctor who was certified by "The American Board of Breast Enhancement Surgery." It sounded impressive until I found out that this board certification could be obtained by attending a weekend course. She was obviously shocked and wished she had understood this doctor's credentials before undergoing her breast implant surgery. It would have prevented her from having to have a secondary operation to correct her deformed breasts.

If you are not sure of the validity of your doctor's board certification, you can research it by contacting The American Board of Medical Specialties (ABMS). The ABMS is considered the gold standard for recognizing which boards are valid due to the intensive training and testing needed to pass these boards. If you look on the ABMS website (www. ABMS.org) you will see that the only valid board for plastic surgeons is The American Board of Plastic Surgery. To be board-certified by The American Board of Plastic Surgery, a physician had to complete at least 5 years of residency training after 4 years of medical school. Once out in practice, an in-depth written examination must be passed. Then, if a plastic surgeon has shown competence in plastic surgery for over a year, the surgeon will then be "grilled" during an extensive oral examination. If the written and oral exams are passed, the board certification will be awarded.

CHAPTER 4

The Nine Biggest Mistakes Patients Make in Plastic Surgery and How to Avoid Them

If you've been considering plastic surgery, your selection of the surgeon may be one of the most important decisions you'll ever make. Making the right choice requires a certain amount of knowledge about the procedures as well as knowing what questions to ask to see if he or she is properly qualified to sculpt your face or body. In addition, you must find your own personal level of comfort and trust with the doctor you select. This chapter will help you in that process and assist you in making the right choice so that you will have the best chance of getting the result you want.

Mistake 1: Not Knowing Where to Start Looking

Once you have decided on a procedure you're interested in, you will want to start compiling a list of doctors to see. Do not just assume that because someone has slick marketing ads that he or she must be good. Marketing should just introduce you to the physician, but not be your sole determining factor in selecting a surgeon. Friends, family, hair stylists, aestheticians, nurses, physicians, or online reviews are all good referral sources. Then, you can start narrowing your list by researching providers by evaluating their training, experience, and credentials. Speaking to an actual patient is also very helpful.

Mistake 2: Choosing Your Surgeon Without Evaluating Training and Credentials

In order for someone to be a "true" plastic surgeon in the United States, they would have to complete four years of an accredited medical school followed by at least three years of general surgery (or some other surgical training) and at least two more years of plastic surgery residency training. However, with diminishing insurance reimbursement, many physicians trained in other fields have taken "short cuts" in their training and called themselves "cosmetic" surgeons. Legally, any doctor can market cosmetic services regardless of their training or competence. They may also make the claim to be "board certified," but it depends on which "board" they are referring to as to whether or not that is of value to you. Some doctors have even gone to a weekend course and gotten some sort of "board certification." Therefore, for the average consumer, deciphering credentials can be confusing and frustrating. Buyer beware!

To find out if a physician's board certification is a valid one, you can log on to the American Board of Medical Specialties website (www.ABMS.org) and view the medical specialty of interest. For example, for plastic surgery, it is critical that your surgeon have board certification by the American Board of Plastic Surgery. Without proper board certification, you have very little assurance that your doctor has completed the rigorous training needed to safely perform surgery. A common "board certification" used by cosmetic surgeons is the "American Board of Cosmetic Surgery." The American Board of Medical Specialties does not recognize this certification because it does not meet their high standards of what constitutes true board certification in a specialty.

In addition, you may want to ask about memberships in medical societies and if the physician has privileges to perform surgery at any accredited facilities in your area.

Mistake 3: Choosing a Surgeon With Whom You Don't Feel Comfortable

When choosing a surgeon, you should feel comfortable discussing your concerns and know that your doctor is listening to you and addressing your desires. Without good communication, it is unlikely that you will obtain the results you want. If the initial consultation seems rushed and the doctor does not seem to have time to answer your questions, then you should consider going elsewhere and getting another opinion. Always remember that surgery is not a one-time event. There will be follow-up visits so you need to take into account that you are entering into a somewhat long-term relationship with a physician you should trust and have good rapport. This will help you with the emotional ups and downs that can follow any surgical procedure. Therefore, be sure your plastic surgeon's office is customer service-oriented and respectful. Above all, be sure they have a good understanding of your desires and expectations.

Mistake 4: Forgetting to Ask About Complications

All procedures have risks associated with them and it is important for you to have an understanding of these risks in order to make an informed decision. Do not be afraid to ask the surgeon about risks and potential complications. In addition, be sure they spend a sufficient amount of time going over your pre and post-operative instructions, consent forms, medications, and expected recovery so that you will have a clear understanding of all the factors involved.

Mistake 5: Getting Surgery for the Wrong Reasons

Some people go through difficult, stressful times and somehow feel that plastic surgery will correct the other difficulties they may have in life. Though plastic surgery may allow you to face the challenges in your life with greater confidence, it should not be viewed as a guarantee that it will fix interpersonal relationship problems. For example, one scenario would be a person who wants to change their appearance because their "significant other" has left them for someone else. Their hope is that by changing their appearance, they may get the love of their life back. Obviously, this may or may not help their relationship problems. Others may think that by changing their appearance, they will be able to get a better job. Therefore, make sure you are correctly motivated and emotionally ready before undergoing any procedure. In addition, be sure no one is pressuring you to have a procedure you really don't want, or don't want right now. Though other people may be glad you are having the procedure, the basic desire needs to come from within yourself.

Patients that do the best are basically happy with themselves, but have a physical feature they would like to improve. They have realistic goals and comply with instructions given for their recovery.

Mistake 6: Forgetting to Ask If You Are a Good Candidate For the Procedure

During a consultation, you and your doctor may get so focused on the problem at hand that you forget to step back and analyze whether or not you are medically a good candidate for surgery. Many patients have underlying health problems that may prohibit them from getting surgery or put them at high risk for complications. Be sure you and your surgeon review all your pertinent medical history before you decide to have a procedure performed. Occasionally, you may be asked to see your primary doctor for a pre-operative clearance to be sure your medical conditions are under good control. The goal should always to provide the safest care for you.

Mistake 7: Choosing Your Surgeon Solely on Price

Having surgery is not like buying a car in which the goal is to get the lowest price. You are paying for a service, not a product. Though all cars of a certain model may be created essentially the same, not all surgeons are equal (please refer to section on credentials above). Though cost certainly is a factor, it should not be the main deciding factor. In life, there is the old saying "You get what you pay for" and plastic surgery is no different. Top quality and highly skilled care at a discount price do not exist. If you are getting a very low price, there must be a reason. No matter how you look at it, higher quality and skill always costs more. By reading this book, we hope you will have a greater understanding of what factors are important so that you will be able to make a more informed decision about your health care. It is hardly a bargain to have a procedure done by an unqualified surgeon and then need a secondary procedure to correct the errors made in the first procedure. You could easily end up paying more than double the cost than if you had made the proper physician choice to start with. Plus, there is the pain and additional time off work associated with a second procedure. Also bear in mind that your highest chance of getting the best result is typically with the first procedure; not a secondary revision.

Mistake 8: Failing to Explore All Your Payment Options

With the ever-increasing acceptance and demand for plastic surgery, many patients want to finance their procedures. Many forget that they can get a home equity loan and the interest rates would be lower than if they resorted to other options. Also, the interest you pay may be tax deductible (ask your accountant for details). Competitive rate credit cards are also a fast and easy option. Another option could be affordable monthly payments arranged through a company, which specifically caters to those interested in cosmetic surgery. Ask your plastic surgeon's office for details on how to finance your procedure.

Mistake 9: Failing to Ask the Right Questions During Your Consultation

There are many questions that will arise during your consultation, some of which are being covered in this book. Many important points are not always covered by the plastic surgeon, so in the next chapter I have listed some questions that are important to ask if the points are not covered in your consultation.

If you avoid these common mistakes listed above, your chance of having a good outcome will be much greater. In addition, you will be better prepared mentally and emotionally to undergo any procedure.

CHAPTER 5

Important Questions to Ask During Your Consultation

Many important points are not always covered by the plastic surgeon during your consultation. Below I have listed some questions that are important to ask if the points are not covered in your consultation.

Is there a consultation fee?

Many surgeons don't tell you there is a fee until after they have completed the consult. Others may claim that the consult is "free" because whatever you paid for the consult is credited towards your surgery.

What is my diagnosis?

In other words, if your physician cannot verbalize and explain to you what is aesthetically not quite right with your face or body, then how can he or she correct the problem? For example, if your breasts are droopy or have an unattractive shape, your surgeon should be able to explain to you if you have ptosis, psuedoptosis, tuberous breasts, constricted breasts, hypoplasia, hyperplasia, inframammary fold asymmetry, etc. Without the basic knowledge of proper diagnosis, then your chances of getting the result you want are very slim. In addition, does the doctor detect any asymmetries in your face and body? Most people are not symmetric and not recognizing that before surgery may lead to a suboptimal result.

Are there any other options to correct my problem?

Your physician should inform you of other options that are available, even if they are not offered in their office. Your doctor should also be willing to refer you to someone else if they don't feel completely competent to perform your procedure.

Have you ever had another patient with my particular situation? If so, how many of these types of procedures have you done?

No physician is an expert at all types of plastic surgery problems. Therefore, it is important for you to be able to evaluate whether or not your doctor has the proper experience and expertise you need.

Can you show me before and after photos of someone who had the procedures you recommend for me?

If a picture is worth a thousand words, then before and after photos should be able to demonstrate the desired result. When you look at the photos, try to imagine if that were you in the photos. Ask yourself if the results look natural or not.

Are these photos of _your_ patients?

Unfortunately, some plastic surgeons will copy photos off another surgeon's website or purchase photos and use them for demonstration purposes. Make sure to ask if the doctor actually did the procedures on the patients in the photos.

Where will my surgery take place?

For surgical procedures, which require sedation or general anesthesia, you will want to be sure that the facility is properly accredited. Accreditation indicates that certain standards for safety are met. Look for accreditation from one of the following national organizations: American Association for Accreditation of Ambulatory Surgical Facilities (AAAASF), Joint Commission on Accreditation of Healthcare Organizations (JCAHO), Accreditation Association for Ambulatory Health Care (AAAHC).

Who will administer my anesthesia?

Most plastic surgery offices only have certified registered nurse anesthetists (CRNA's) administering the anesthesia. Others will provide a board-certified anesthesiologist (who is an M.D.), which is considered the highest level of anesthetic care for you. Therefore, be sure to ask about the credentials of your anesthesia provider.

What will my recovery be like?

When undergoing surgery, it is important to have an understanding of the expected recuperation. You will be more at ease after the procedure if you know that the things you are going through are "normal." In addition, you may need to take some time off of work and have others take care of domestic issues, such as laundry, yard work, housecleaning, etc. Your plastic surgeon's office should not only review the post-operative expectations, medications, and scar care with you in advance, they should also give you written information that describes your recovery.

What are the risks involved in my procedure?

All procedures carry some level of risk. It is important for you to be able to understand those risks and how they would be handled if a complication occurred. Your plastic surgeon's office should not only explain the risks verbally, they should also provide you with written information at least one week before your procedure so that you will be able to make the best decision with respect to your healthcare.

What happens if I have a complication, which requires a secondary procedure?

Though none of us likes to think of the chances of having complications, they are a fact of life in an imperfect world. Everything in life has some risk attached and while we are on planet Earth, there will always be unfortunate situations that arise. Be sure to ask about their revision policy so there won't be any undesirable surprises if a complication arises.

Will my health insurance cover any facility or anesthesia fees if I should have a complication and need additional surgery?

All insurance plans vary. You would need to check your own policy for coverage.

Should I talk with any former patients who have had this procedure?

If you need further explanation from a patient's perspective, it may be worthwhile talking to a former patient. They may offer valuable information that may have not been covered in your consultation. However, remember that patients are private individuals and respect for their time is appreciated.

CHAPTER 6

Body Contouring – Liposuction, Tummy Tucks and Other Lifting Procedures

Despite a healthy diet and an exercise routine, many men and women are frustrated with the inability to eliminate stubborn fat that doesn't want to go away in the waist, upper abdomen, hips, back, or other areas. Sometimes the figure generally looks good, but there is a disproportionate localized accumulation of fat in certain areas.

After having children or major weight loss, there are physical changes to the body, especially after multiple births. The abdomen stretches, there may be stretch marks and loose skin, and there can be a ballooning of the abdomen. I also frequently see patients that have had a significant reduction in weight and they have loose, hanging skin all around their body, including from the neck as well as the arms, legs, and thighs.

We have solutions to these concerns that include removal of excess fat accumulations from problematic areas through liposuction and in some cases we will additionally tighten the abdomen and remove excess loose skin with an abdominoplasty, or what is commonly known as a "tummy tuck." We also have lifting procedures that can address loose skin on the neck, arms, thighs and legs.

Body Contouring with Liposuction

When we are talking about contouring the body, the most common and well-known technique used is liposuction, which is suction-assisted fat removal. Hundreds of thousands of liposuction cases are performed in America every year. We typically use liposuction to remove fat accumulations from the abdomen, the flanks, or "love handles," the back, and thighs. We can also use liposuction to remove fat from the arms and breasts.

Liposuction technology has developed over the past few decades and, as plastic surgeons, we have a number of techniques available to improve the results and minimize recovery time. Some of these advances have included the use of lasers or ultrasound in combination with liposuction to assist with fat removal.

I have researched the various liposuction techniques as they have been developed and I have found that the best results, minimizing bruising and recovery time, are achieved with the combination of three techniques: "tumescent technique," "laser-assisted," and "power-assisted liposuction."

With the "tumescent technique," a saline solution with a local anesthesia and a small amount of adrenaline is injected into the fat to shrink the blood vessels, which leads to less bleeding and bruising. For smaller volume cases we can perform the liposuction while the patient is awake. For cases where a larger volume of fat is being removed, we will put the patient to sleep with an IV anesthesia and then inject the fat with the tumescent fluid.

Next, I use a laser-assisted technique by applying an Erchonia® laser to the fat to soften it for easier removal. The Erchonia laser is a cold laser that is applied to the exterior of the body at the area being treated and it penetrates the skin and fat with laser energy. This allows removal of more fat especially in dense areas such as the upper back, upper abdomen, or chest areas.

There are alternative laser techniques used by other plastic surgeons that use a hot laser inserted through an incision under the skin to melt the fat. However, this heat could be transmitted to the skin and burn it, which would lead to undesirable, visible, permanent scarring. These technologies were originally intended for small cases that could be done under local anesthesia, with the patient awake. There are claims that use of the hot laser can shrink the skin, but the only way to shrink skin is by passing the laser just under the skin from the inside, causing a mild internal burn of the skin. This will cause the heat to transfer to the skin and therefore make the collagen shrink. Unfortunately, this technique is fraught with problems because any minor imperfection in the technique will result in dimpling, depressions, grooves, or possibly burns and scarring in the skin. Some people have had chronic burning sensations after hot lasers have been used. Seromas, or fluid accumulations under the skin, are also possible.

I have chosen not to use the hot laser technique because the Erchonia laser technology is far superior, gives better results, decreases downtime, and has no risk of complications. The Erchonia laser is a "cold" laser so there has never been even one case of a burn.

After the Erchonia laser application, I use power-assisted liposuction to remove the fat. Traditional liposuction works by forcefully and quickly "ramming" a metal tube (called a "cannula") into the fat to break it up while a vacuum is applied to remove the fat. This type of liposuction is fairly traumatic and has been associated with internal organ injuries. In contrast, power-assisted liposuction uses a smaller diameter cannula, which is mounted on a special handpiece that causes the cannula to vibrate back and forth just a fraction of an inch at a very high speed—thousands of times per minute. This back and forth action breaks up the fat in a gentler manner. The vibration also causes some internal shrinkage of the tissues that helps shrink up the skin as well.

The handpiece can be held with two fingers and slowly is passed into the fat layer in a slow, rhythmic fashion.

Therefore, the chance of internal organ damage is virtually eliminated because as long as the cannula is in the fatty layer, it glides easily; if the cannula reaches the muscle, it becomes hard to advance it. If it becomes hard to advance, we simply stop the advancement of the cannula, back up, and head off in a different direction.

Liposuction Frequently Asked Questions

Can't I just diet or exercise more to lose the fat?

Some people, even though they regularly exercise and maintain a healthy diet, have certain areas that have excess fat that they can't seem to lose. With weight reduction through diet and exercise, as you lose weight, you don't really change your shape significantly. You become a smaller version of the same shape, whereas with liposuction we can permanently change the shape and make the curves more aesthetically pleasing. Genetically, sometimes people hang on to fat in certain areas and can't get rid of it. The most common areas of concern are the "love handles," or flanks, the abdomen, and for women, the outer thighs.

You cannot spot reduce fat by working the muscle in a certain area. As an example, exercising the thigh muscles doesn't reduce the fat in the thigh. Fat loss doesn't work like that; the thigh muscle doesn't preferentially grab energy from the fat in your thigh. When losing weight from exercise or diet, all the fat cells in the body get a little bit smaller, so that's where liposuction is oftentimes superior to just weight loss, as it can specifically reduce the fat and contour the shape in the area of concern.

Is the fat removed from liposuction permanently removed?

Yes, the fat is permanently removed with liposuction. The amount of human fat cells is set during childhood and stays the same during our adult lives. Since liposuction removes fat cells, those cells removed with liposuction are gone forever.

When should I be able to see the results?

Patients will notice the difference right away, but because the fat is fragile and easy to suction out, it also means that that tissue tends to swell significantly. Usually in about five to seven days after surgery, patients notice significant amount of swelling. Now they're typically not bigger than they were before the surgery, but they go through this period where they may look at themselves in the mirror and wonder if the surgery was really worth it? A month or so later, they can start seeing a significant body contour change.

At three months, at least 80% of the swelling is gone and the remaining 20% of the swelling can take six months to a year to go away completely. We often follow up with patients up to a year post-op and if we take photographs of them, and as long as they haven't gained weight, then you can very clearly observe a difference between the three-month photos and the one-year photos.

How much weight can I lose with liposuction?

We explain to our patients that liposuction is mainly a contouring procedure and it's not considered a weight-loss procedure. When we do liposuction, there is a limit to how much fat we can safely remove in one day. Typically we would limit the amount of liposuction in a day to removing about 5 to 6 liters of fat, which translates into about 11 to 13 pounds. The difference in liposuction and regular weight loss is that when you lose 11 to 13 pounds through diet or exercise, all your fat cells from head to toe get a little bit smaller. With liposuction, you're spot reducing that weight in areas that are bothersome. People can lose 10 pounds with liposuction and look like they've lost 25 pounds with just normal weight loss through exercise or diet.

Once I've lost the fat cells with liposuction, can I forget about my diet and exercise and still maintain my new figure?

We coach our patients into making some lifestyle changes after their surgery (see Chapter 16). We can contour and take away fat and sculpt the shape, making patients look great. However, if they don't maintain their body, they could lose their results. The vast majority of my patients have gone on to actually lose a little bit more weight on their own. We educate them on a healthy lifestyle, psychologically they're encouraged, and with liposuction, we have changed the muscle-to-fat ratio in the body.

The muscle is the engine that burns the fat and that hasn't changed. If there are fewer fat cells in the body, now the muscle-to-fat ratio is more in their favor. Even if they maintain the same exercise plan they were doing before, now there are fewer fat cells to burn up so that they tend to lose a little bit more weight after the surgery. If there is a weight gain after liposuction, we typically will see the calories will follow the path of least resistance. So let's say a woman had a major amount of liposuction of her abdomen, her flanks, her legs, and then she puts on weight. The path of least resistance would typically dictate that the fat would go first to the breasts and then to the buttocks and then wherever else fat cells can be found. It might come back in places that she's not accustomed to gaining weight when she puts back on weight.

How long until I can go back to work and resume normal activities?

Depending on how many areas are treated, most patients get back to work in a week or less. We encourage patients to wait two weeks before resuming exercise and to try to limit salt intake in order to avoid excessive swelling. Since fat is a fragile organ, it tends to swell after the surgery. About half the swelling is resolved in the first month. The rest of the swelling can take three to twelve months to resolve completely. Patients are sore for a few days with diminishing discomfort for 2 to 4 weeks depending on the volume removed.

Will I have to wear a compressive garment after surgery?

Yes. Careful measurements will be taken to provide you with a compressive garment that will help minimize your swelling. Ideally, you would wear the garment at least 20 hours per day for the first three weeks. After that, we recommend you wear the garment at least 12 hours per day (or night) for the next two months.

Tummy Tuck (Abdominoplasty)

A "tummy tuck," also known as "abdominoplasty," removes excess abdominal skin and tightens deep abdominal muscles. The improvement in contour can be quite dramatic, with better fitting clothes, even getting back into a bathing suit when you never thought you would. Abdominoplasty helps to improve the contour of the abdomen and to narrow the waist by tightening the abdominal muscles. Women with stretched abdominal areas due to pregnancies or men with major weight loss can benefit considerably from abdominoplasty. Other individuals, whose skin has lost some of its elasticity and are slightly obese, can also experience an improvement in their abdominal area with this procedure.

When doing a consultation for fat removal in the abdomen with liposuction, we make an assessment whether we think that the skin will be saggy when we're finished with the liposuction procedure. There are some variables that determine the ability for the skin to retract itself. The age of the patient makes a significant difference because once we break the age barrier of around thirty-five years old, skin starts to lose elasticity fairly quickly. We also examine the thickness and the quality of the existing skin. Genetically, some people have very loose skin to begin with, and their skin is not going to retract as well as patients with thicker, sturdier skin. If we see stretch marks, the skin has been damaged beyond its ability to repair itself, and there will not be significant skin retraction with laser or liposuction. Our examination will provide an indication of the outcome of the liposuction procedure and if we expect that the result will not achieve what the patient is looking for, we try to warn them ahead of time that they may want to go ahead and have a tummy tuck at the same time.

People that have lost a large amount of weight, say over 50 pounds, or women that have had children, often have a separation in the vertical "six-pack" muscles in the abdomen. The weight gain and loss has stretched the muscles beyond their ability to repair themselves. Even after the weight loss, the abdomen balloons, and no matter how much you work those muscles, you'll never end up with a flat abdomen again. This would be another indicator that would influence our decision to encourage the patient to have a tummy tuck.

The tummy tuck will not only remove the loose, saggy skin, but internally we stitch the muscles back together where they used to be before pregnancy or the weight gain/loss. This tightens the muscles up so the patient can have a flat abdomen again. Some patients, even if they don't have loose skin, still get a tummy tuck to tighten up their muscles and regain the flat abdomen.

Depending on your aesthetic goals and degree of abdominal skin laxity, there are several tummy tuck options. The simplest tummy tuck, with the least amount of scarring, is the "mini-tummy tuck." Patients without much skin laxity or who just need their abdominal muscles tightened are good candidates for this procedure. A short incision will be placed within the swimsuit area and stitches are placed in 1 or 2 layers to bring the rectus ("six pack") muscles back to the midline to tighten and flatten the abdomen. Also, with the mini-tummy tuck, the belly button can be moved down about an inch from the inside without creating an external scar. (NOTE: some plastic surgeons do not repair the rectus muscles with the mini-tummy tuck. Be sure to ask for details before you commit to a procedure.)

If the skin has more laxity requiring more skin removal, then the scar must be made longer and a "standard tummy tuck," or "classic tummy tuck" will be indicated. An incision is made in the lower abdomen within your swimsuit area and the skin is dissected up to the ribs. If a muscle repair is needed, then stitches are placed in 1 or 2 layers to bring the rectus muscles back to the midline to tighten and flatten the abdomen. The skin is then re-draped down under some tension and the excess skin is removed. The belly-button stalk is also freed up so that it won't end up too low. Once the excess skin is removed, a new "hole" is created and the belly button brought out through that hole and stitched into place.

When patients lose large amounts of weight, for example over 100 pounds, they are likely good candidates for an "extended tummy tuck," which has a longer hip-to-hip scar, or a "circumferential tummy tuck," which is also called a "lower body lift." In this case the scar goes all the way around the lower body and not only tightens the midsection, it also lifts the outer thighs and buttocks. The final option for patients with excessively loose skin in both the vertical and horizontal dimensions is to combine their tummy tuck with a "vertical skin removal" procedure.

After a typical tummy tuck, the raw area between the undersurface of the skin and the muscles will weep a dilute bloody fluid. We put one or two drains in the abdominal area and there are suction bulbs at the end of the tubes to drain out the fluid. The drains typically are removed in 2 to 3 weeks after the procedure. One issue for patients is that the bulbs are difficult to hide.

I also perform an advanced tummy tuck procedure known as the "Hollywood Tummy Tuck," where we stitch the skin internally to the muscles in multiple areas, thereby eliminating the space where the dilute bloody fluid would normally accumulate. With this procedure drains are not needed. This procedure takes about 30-45 minutes longer because of the additional stitching. The down side of the Hollywood tummy tuck is that temporarily, until those internal stitches dissolve, the patient is going to see some dents in the abdominal skin because the skin has being sewn down to the muscle. Those dents can take anywhere from one to three months to go away completely, so if you're planning a summer vacation in a month or two, you may not want to get the Hollywood tummy tuck.

Tummy Tuck Frequently Asked Questions

What kind of scar am I going to be left with? Will it be visible when I wear a swimsuit?

The residual scarring with a tummy tuck is probably the number one concern expressed by patients during their consultation. The length of the tummy tuck scar is determined by how much skin we can remove vertically. In very rough terms imagine a piece of skin removed in the shape of a football. The taller the football gets, the longer the football gets, as well. For patients without much skin removal, the scar will be very short, maybe six inches. If the patient has a lot of skin removed, then it can easily be a hip-to-hip scar.

The goal of the surgery is to be able to hide the scar in a swimsuit. I always insist that my patients bring in a swimsuit that they want to wear after surgery on the day of surgery. I mark the swimsuit on their body and they can be guaranteed that the scar will be hidden. No matter what swimsuit style they bring in, whether it's a horizontal low swimsuit or the kind that makes your legs look longer by arching up toward the hips, we can make the scar land within the swimsuit without any problem. It's not the length of the scar that's as important as the location of the scar. If it's properly placed, women will end up back in a two-piece swimsuit.

How do I know if liposuction is needed with my tummy tuck?

Often tummy tucks are done in combination with liposuction of various areas such as the abdomen, flanks (or "muffin top"), back, thighs, or arms in order to give a more harmonious improvement in contours. Combining these procedures not only improves the overall end result, it also saves money and allows for only one recovery period instead of two.

Would a tummy tuck typically be done at the same time as the liposuction?

Yes, we typically do the liposuction at the same time as the tummy tuck. With the advancements in liposuction, it is very safe to do both together and it helps patients to get it all done at one time so they can save money and have only one recovery, with less time off of work.

Is a tummy tuck a permanent fix?

The results do tend to be permanent. I've even had some patients that were still significantly heavy when they had their tummy tucks and did not want to have a gastric bypass. They had the tummy tuck to eliminate overhanging skin that they had that was bothering them. After the surgery they were encouraged and went on to lose 50 to 80 pounds and they did not lose the result of the tummy tuck even though they subsequently lost a lot of weight.

When can I return to work and resume normal activities?

After a tummy tuck, patients usually are able to return to work in two weeks. Although we encourage light activity right away, we recommend patients wait at least three weeks before resuming vigorous exercise and to try to limit salt intake in order to avoid excessive swelling. There is some swelling after the surgery; about half the swelling is resolved in the first month. The rest of the swelling can take approximately six to twelve months to resolve completely.

Will I have to wear a compressive garment after surgery?

Yes. Careful measurements will be taken to provide you with an abdominal binder right after surgery. After one to two weeks, you will then transition to a compressive garment that will help minimize your swelling. Ideally, you would wear the binder or garment at least 12 to 18 hours per day for the first three weeks. We recommend you remove the binder when you are in bed to reduce the pressure on your leg veins. After three weeks, we recommend you wear the garment at least 12 hours per day for the next two months.

Other Lifting Procedures

There are a number of lifting procedures that are commonly performed to address specific patient concerns. Facelifts can reduce the signs of aging by removing excess fat, tightening the underlying muscle and re-draping the skin around the neck and face. For patients that have excess skin hanging from the neck, I perform a more conservative procedure known as a "neck lift".

In Chapter 11, about body contouring after major weight loss, I describe a number of other lifting procedures to address loose skin in the arms, legs, thighs, and in cases of a major weight loss, more extensive procedures to address loose skin around the entire midsection.

Patient History: 32 year old who underwent laser-assisted liposuction of hips and outher thighs. After photo is 3 months post-op.

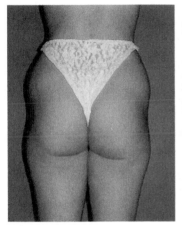 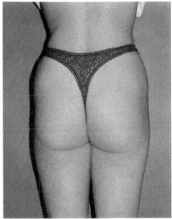

Patient History: 38 Year old who underwent laser-assisted liposuction of her abdomen, upper back, and flanks. After photos are 3 months post-op.

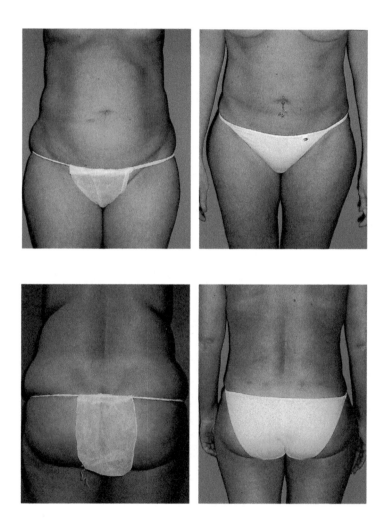

Patient History: 30 Year old female who underwent Brazillian Butt Lift. After photos are 3 months post-op.

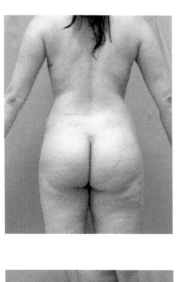 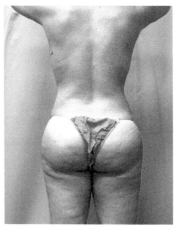

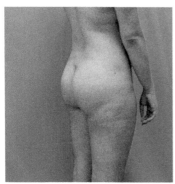 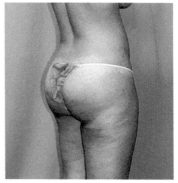

CHAPTER 7

Breast Augmentation

Breast augmentation is among the most commonly performed cosmetic surgery procedures in the world today. Either silicone or saline-filled implants are inserted either under the crease of the breast, around the areola, or through the armpit. Your implants can be placed under the breast tissue or beneath the main chest (pectoral) muscle. Our goal with breast augmentation is to create beautiful breasts that look natural and give the size and look that the patient wants. After surgery, your breasts will appear fuller and shapelier and the incision scars will fade over time.

Under ideal circumstances, any elective surgery would result in minimal discomfort and a speedy recovery. Though it is not really possible to have absolutely no discomfort after surgery, the techniques I use now make it possible to minimize your discomfort after procedure and return to normal activities sooner. Over the years and after thousands of cases, I have perfected the breast augmentation procedure and we now call it our "Quick Recovery Breast Augmentation."

When most surgeons perform breast augmentations, they typically utilize blunt trauma techniques to create the pocket, which will accommodate the implant. As a result, there is bleeding and bruising of the tissues which causes more inflammation and therefore more pain. Our technique starts weeks before the surgery ever begins. First, we educate patients as to the nutritional supplements they can begin taking preoperatively to help their bodies heal faster. Second, local anesthetics are injected after the patient is put to sleep, but before the surgery begins. This allows the surgery to be done with less intravenous medications which results in a decreased inflammatory response to the surgery. This also leads to less discomfort. Third, I perform the surgery without blunt trauma, but rather careful and precise creation of the pockets for the implants with meticulous attention to stop any bleeding. Excess blood left in the pockets will cause more irritation of the tissues and lead to more inflammation and more soreness. At the end of the procedure, local anesthesia is either sprayed into the pocket to assist with post-op discomfort (which lasts for a few hours), or if you choose, a new long-acting local anesthetic (Exparel) can be injected during surgery that lasts much longer. Exparel will numb up the area where it is injected and alleviate pain for 1 to 3 days. Another option would be a pain pump that uses very small tubes (catheters) to pump anesthesia into the internal wound are for 3-5 days. Exparel and pain pumps do not cause sedation so you can be alert and have your pain controlled. As a result, many of our patients do not need to use any narcotic pain medications, thus avoiding the potential side effects of those drugs, and enjoying a quicker and more pleasant recovery.

We also encourage light activity to keep the muscles from becoming stiff and uncomfortable. A light, compressive Ace wrap and bra are placed at the end of the case to further reduce your post-operative swelling and tenderness. We encourage our patients to return to non-strenuous activity within 24 hours of their surgery. Most of our patients typically say that the procedure was much easier than they ever thought it would be and highly recommend it to other women. Their only regret is that they didn't do it sooner so they could enjoy the benefits of their appearance longer!

Implant Placement Under the Muscle vs. Above the Muscle

One of the decisions a patient must make is whether to have the implants placed under or over the pectoral muscle. During patient consultation we provide information to assist patients in making the decision that best suits their aesthetic goals and lifestyles.

Subglandular implant Subpectoral implant

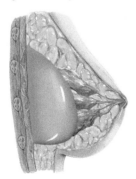 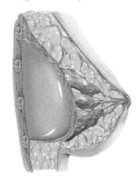

The **BENEFITS** of having the implants under the muscle ("submuscular") include:

1) Saline implants typically look better under the muscle ("submuscular") because there is more coverage of the upper part of the implant, which tends to hide the edge of the implant. Also, saline implants have a higher tendency to show visible rippling and the pectoral muscle can minimize the visibility of the rippling in the cleavage area. The muscle does not cover the lateral or inferior aspects of the implant (i.e. technically called "partial submuscular") and therefore, rippling may be visible in these areas. Silicone implants can be put under or over the muscle and look good in either position.

2) Mammograms are slightly better with submuscular implants.

3) The capsular contracture rate is slightly lower for submuscular implants when compared to implants put under the breast gland ("sub glandular"). However, if the implants are placed in the subfacial plane over the muscle, then the capsular contracture rate is almost the same as under the muscle placement. (Dissection into the subfascial plane is achieved by lifting the tough fibrous fascia layer off the pectoral muscle along with the breast gland.) In some women who don't work out their pectoral muscles, the pectoral muscle can help hold the weight of the implant so the tendency to sag should be less. However, if you do a lot of chest

exercises, this can actually cause the implants to drift laterally and inferiorly over time.

The **DISADVANTAGES** of having the implants placed under the muscle include:

1) The post-op recovery is more painful because the muscle gets stretched. As a result, we recommend you consider getting the injections of a long-acting anesthetic (Exparel) or a pain pump placed at the time of surgery, as described above. Exparel or pain pumps will numb up the area where it is injected and alleviate your pain for about 3 days. Exparel or pain pumps do not cause sedation so you can be alert and have your pain controlled. As a result, many of our patients do not need to use any narcotic pain medications, thus avoiding the potential side effects of those drugs, and enjoying a quicker and more pleasant recovery.

2) The implants get pulled up by the pectoral muscle and ride high for up to three months.

3) Whenever the pectoral muscle is flexed (even in daily activities such as lifting grocery bags), your breasts will move with the muscle. Some women find this breast animation disturbing and unnatural. In addition, it sometimes brings unwanted attention and questions regarding why their breasts move in that manner.

4) For women that like to do upper body exercises such as weight lifting, resistance training, Yoga, Pilates, push ups, bench press, chest flyes, etc., the pectoral muscle can stretch out the implant pocket over time and cause your implants to drift laterally and downward. To

repair this, the implants must be removed, the implant pocket adjusted with multiple internal stitches, and a new pocket created above the muscle in the subfascial plane. In addition, some women also need removal of excessive breast skin (i.e. breast lift) at the same time in order to regain a normal shape. This would lead to breast scarring. Therefore, for athletic women who want to continue doing chest exercises, we typically recommend that the implants be placed above the muscle in the subfascial plane as long as there is enough upper breast fullness to cover the implants and not risk visible rippling. We also recommend silicone implants for above-the-muscle subfascial placement because they have a more natural look and feel with less tendency than saline implants to show visible rippling. For those who choose subfascial augmentation, we do not recommend the injection of Exparel or pain pumps because they are not necessary.

The **BENEFITS** of having implants placed above the muscle (subfascial placement) include:

1) Less pain. For this procedure, it is not necessary for you to get the Exparel injection option mentioned above. Patients typically go back to work in a few days verses about a week for submuscular augmentation patients.

2) Quicker recovery. When the implants are placed above the muscle, the muscle does not lift the implant, as is the case with submuscular placement. Therefore, the implants have "settled" into their natural position soon after surgery.

3) With implants above the muscle, there is minimal animation of the breasts with flexion of the pectoral muscle.

4) With implants above the muscle, you can perform heavy chest exercises without dislodging the implants.

5) Breast implants above the muscle tend to be somewhat softer than below the muscle because in the submuscular position, the pectoral muscle tone can exert constant tension on the implant making it feel firmer.

6) The fascia above the pectoral muscle is a strong sheet of connective tissue. Therefore, if we put your implants in the subfascial plane, this will act like an internal bra to help keep your implants from dropping over time.

Saline vs. Silicone Gel Implants

In the 1990's, there was some controversy as to the safety of silicone gel implants. The media portrayed silicone implants as toxic substances that were ruining women's lives. Dow Corning decided on a $4 billion settlement instead of trying to fight the lawsuits. The FDA restricted first-time augmentation patients from getting silicone gel. However, what most people don't realize is that the FDA did not completely ban silicone gel implants from the market. For example, if a woman had saline implants that rippled, she could get them exchanged for silicone implants; if a woman needed a breast lift along with augmentation, she could opt for silicone implants; and if a woman had breast cancer and needed reconstruction after mastectomy, she could choose silicone implants. So, you must ask yourself, if the

FDA thought silicone implants were dangerous, then why would they allow them in cancer patients? You should also ask yourself why the United States was the only country in the world to put a ban on silicone implants. The story is long and convoluted involving political and financial gain. The implant companies repeated all their safety studies, and in 2006 the FDA re-approved silicone gel implants for women over 22 years old. They found no link between silicone implants and disease or cancer. Premier Plastic Surgery Center was one of the offices that was allowed to use silicone implants during the years they were "banned." We submitted our data to the FDA, which helped get the silicone implants re-approved for general use. Prior to 2006, about 35% of our patients chose silicone implants. (All of these patients entered into the FDA's breast implant study.) Now, over 90% of our patients choose silicone implants because of the more natural look and feel.

The largest benefit of silicone implants over saline is that they look and feel more natural. Even though the implants are round, they take on more of a teardrop shape when compared to the saline implants. For small-breasted women, this is particularly important. In addition, silicone implants look good under or over the pectoral muscle (see above for details). You could also choose to have anatomic ("teardrop") shaped "gummy bear" implants placed, which have less upper breast fullness (i.e. a softer slope) compared to the "plump" look of round implants.

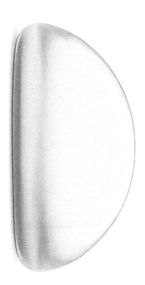 

Round Silicone
Gel Implant

Teardrop "Gummy
Bear" Implant

The main benefits of the saline implants is that the cost is lower and if they ever leak, your body absorbs the fluid making it obvious that you need to have a replacement. If the silicone implant ruptures, it is difficult to diagnose because the breasts look and feel the same due to the new cohesive gel used to fill the implants. You would need the help of a radiologist to detect a leaky silicone implant. For that reason, the FDA has recommended, but not required, that women with silicone implants undergo an MRI scan three years after surgery and every two years after that. The good news is that the new silicone implants have a cohesive gel that tends to stick together and not migrate like the old silicone gel. Migration of the gel could cause the breasts or underarm lymph nodes to become lumpy, but there is no evidence that this caused disease or cancer.

The disadvantages of saline implants are that they tend to show rippling (and therefore typically should be placed under the pectoral muscle); they feel like a bag of water and not a natural breast; and they tend to have more of a round look instead of a teardrop appearance.

Incision Options

As plastic surgeons, we always try to hide scars as well as minimize them. The underarm incision is a great way to hide the scar. When a lot of surgeons use the underarm approach, they take a blunt instrument and rip and tear to create a pocket for the implant. This can cause excessive pain, bruising, slower recovery, increased risk of internal breast bleeding after surgery, and higher risk of capsular contracture. However, I have never used this blunt trauma technique. I have always used endoscopic, or "fiber-optic," scopes with sterile cameras so I can see inside the breast and precisely make the pocket exactly where we want the implant to be placed. We also stop every bleeding blood vessel along the way. Typically, patients lose less than a teaspoon of blood during the procedure. The scars are well hidden along a natural fold in the underarm. At 6-12 months after surgery, most patients cannot find their own scars. We can put any size saline implant through this access, but because silicone gel implants are pre-filled, we usually limit the size of silicone implant that we put through the underarm to approximately 600cc.

For those who want silicone implants larger than 600cc, the next option we recommend would be at the bottom of the breast (inframammary crease). This incision is placed just off the crease and slightly on to the breast in order to avoid scar irritation by the bra. For silicone implants, we routinely use a Keller Funnel in order to reduce the scar length, reduce the risk of infection, and minimize the chance of getting a capsular contracture.

You also have the option to have the incision made around the areola. This resulting scar typically forms a fine line and is placed at the junction of the pigmented areola and lighter-colored breast skin in order to try to hide it. Unfortunately, this access has the disadvantage of having the highest chance of losing nipple sensation, highest infection rate, highest capsular contracture rate, and leads to some decreased milk production.

Breast Augmentation Frequently Asked Questions

Do the implants have any type of warranty?

Yes, the implant companies we use (Sientra, Mentor, and Allergan) all have Lifetime Warranties on the implants for no additional charge. In addition, if they leak in the first ten years, the implant company will also pay you a certain amount of money to help offset the fees you incur to have them replaced. You may purchase an upgraded warranty that will increase the reimbursement level in the first ten years if desired.

Will the implants affect nipple sensation?

Most women have a temporary change in nipple sensation (either more or less sensitive) after augmentation because the sensory nerves have been stretched. The nerves may take 3-12 months to fully recover from the stretch injury. In my experience only a small percentage (1-2%) of women do not recover sensation because either the nerves were stretched so far, they ruptured, or the nerves anatomically were not in the right place and were damaged at the time of surgery. There is no way to tell in advance if you are at risk for losing nipple sensation.

Will I be able to breast feed after augmentation?

Yes. If you choose to have your access incision in the underarm or at the bottom of the breast, then the breast should function normally. If you choose to have the incision around the areola, then some of the ducts may get divided and there will be some decreased milk production, but that will not prevent you from being able to breast feed.

What is a Keller Funnel?

The Keller Funnel is a soft, nylon, disposable triangular "sleeve" (similar to an icing bag) that allows us to insert the silicone gel implants in through a smaller opening and minimize any chance of damaging the implant during its' placement. In addition, the implant never touches the skin during this process. Preliminary data on this device indicate that it may also be effective in reducing the likelihood of infection or developing a capsular contracture.

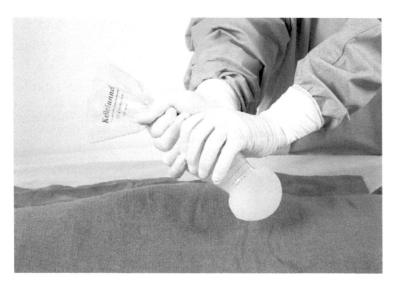

What is Capsular Contracture and how can it be prevented?

Whenever any synthetic device is implanted in a patient, the body will form a scar tissue capsule around the object. The good news is that this scar tissue capsule can help hold the weight of the breast implant and thereby reduce the tendency to droop over time. However, in some women, for reasons we don't fully understand, the scar tissue capsule can shrink and squeeze the implant. We call this a "capsular contracture." If this occurs, the breast will feel firmer and the implant typically takes on the form of a sphere. The capsular contracture can also change the shape or position of the breast implant. Typically, the implants are displaced upward.

Factors that increase the risk of capsular contracture include trauma, bacterial infection, excessive blood or fluid (i.e. "hematoma" or "seroma") in the breast pocket, smoking, and radiation. To prevent capsular contractures, we use meticulous surgical technique to assure complete sterility and insure that there is no bleeding at the end of the case. We also use powder-free gloves, antibiotic irrigation, and a "no touch" technique (the implant never touches the skin or surgical drapes). It is either in its' sterile container or we are inserting it in the patient. Only the surgeon touches the implant, never the scrub tech or nurse. The "cleaner" the implant, the less likely a capsular contracture will form.

Also, patients with smooth implants are instructed on how to do proper breast massages to further minimize the chance of contracture. Vitamin E along with multivitamins has also been shown to be beneficial. Anti-asthma medicines such as Accolate or Singulair have been used with limited success. This would be an "off label" use of these medications, which means the FDA does not have a clear indication for these medications to be used for capsular contracture. Finally, textured implants may reduce the likelihood of capsular contractures, but some studies failed to show any benefit.

At Premier Plastic Surgery Center, we have a very low capsular contracture rate (less than 3%). In addition, we have a laser, which can be used to soften the capsular contractures without performing surgery. Of the few patients that have developed capsular contractures and received laser therapy, over half of them did not need surgical revision because the laser was able to soften the scar tissue capsules.

Are there any Possible Negative Health Issues Associated With Breast Implants?

Millions of women have had breast implants placed over the past 50 years. The vast majority have had no negative side effects. There was controversy in the early 1990's over the safety of silicone implants leading to a partial ban on silicone implants by the FDA. After extensive studies, the FDA released silicone for general use in 2006 after finding that silicone and saline implants had essentially the same complication rates. Many articles have been published over the past 20 years regarding "silicone-induced diseases." Likewise, articles have been published showing that silicone and saline implants are not causing diseases. So, the "jury" is still out. However, there is one entity that no one disputes. Very rarely, patients can have **chronic infection** from a foreign body (breast implant, pacemaker, artificial joint, or any other implanted synthetic object). Germs can live on a foreign body and secrete a "bio-film" which is like an umbrella covering them. Therefore, antibiotics or your own natural immune system cells cannot fight this infection. The germs live on the foreign body and give off their waste products thereby causing a whole host of symptoms such as fatigue, itching, rashes, tingling, joint pain, toxic shock syndrome, insomnia, depression, hair loss, memory loss, headaches, mood swings, etc. The human body will typically detect there is a problem and wall off this infection with layers of scar tissue. This makes it even harder for the immune system cells or antibiotics to attack these germs. Therefore, the only way to clear this type of problem is by removing the foreign body and the surrounding scar tissue capsule. Then the body's immune system is able to clear out the remaining germs because they no longer have the foreign body on which to latch on. However, it is important to emphasize that this may or may not cause the improvement of the symptoms. Also, it may take months or years to fully recuperate from the damage done by the chronic infection.

What can be done if chronic infection or implant-related diseases are suspected?

Though this scenario is extremely rare, some patients have extensive work-ups by their primary care doctor to try to determine the cause of their symptoms. These workups may include blood tests and imaging studies (such as ultrasound, MRI scan, CT scan, etc.).

In the unlikely event that implant and scar tissue removal is necessary, what surgical procedures can be done to remove my implants and the surrounding scar tissue capsule?

There are 2 procedures that can be done. The first procedure is an **implant removal with a capsulectomy**. (A capsulectomy involves removing the entire scar tissue capsule that surrounds the implant.) In this type of surgery, the implant is removed first and then the scar tissue capsule is removed. On the day of surgery, multiple cultures would be sent off to a lab for analysis to see if there are any organisms growing in the breast implant pocket. We also send off the scar tissue for microscopic analysis by a pathologist.

The other operation would be an **En Bloc** procedure. This means that the implant and scar tissue capsule are removed simultaneously as one big "block." This is often done when it is known pre-operatively that a silicone implant has ruptured because it helps contain the "free" silicone inside the scar tissue capsule. An En Bloc removal is rarely done with saline implants. Also, this surgery takes longer than a removal of implants with capsulectomies (therefore more expensive) and requires a much larger opening to get all the contents out in a single block of tissue.

Either surgery above will have a drain in each breast to remove the dilute bloody (serosanguinous) fluid that is generated from the surgical trauma. The drains typically stay in for 1-2 weeks. The recovery for either surgery is about the same. Most women take a week off from a desk job and don't exercise for 3 weeks.

If my implants and scar tissue capsules need to be removed, how soon after they are removed will I start to feel better?

There is no guarantee that removing the implants and scar tissue capsules will improve your health. Since the symptoms women experience tend not to be isolated to the breasts (such as breast pain only), removing the implants may have no benefit in curing total body symptoms. If the symptoms were caused by the implants (such as chronic infection), then patients sometimes start feeling better within 1-3 weeks after surgery. If an infection has been there for years, it could take longer to have a full recovery. If the cultures demonstrated an infection, we would typically refer you to an infectious disease specialist. Some patients have also chosen to have "detox" protocols at physician's offices that deal with "natural healing".

Patient History: 23 year old athletic female who underwent endoscopic tranaxillary (underarm) subfacial (over the muscle) 385cc smooth Allergan silicone breast augmentation. Post-op photos are 3 months after surgery. She went from a 32A cup bra to a 34D.

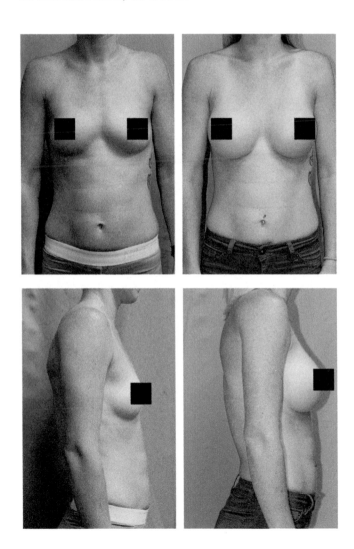

Patient History: 35 year old female who had submuscular smooth Allergan silicone implants (410cc on the right and 380cc on the left). The post-op photo is 3 months after surgery.

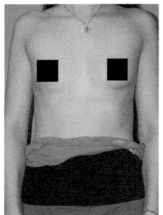 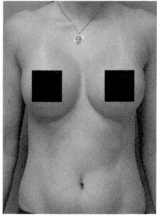

CHAPTER 8

Breast Lift/Mastopexy

Women's breasts can change dramatically over a lifetime due to hormonal changes, pregnancy and breast-feeding, change in weight, loss of elasticity over time, surgery, and gravity. The nipples can also change and the diameter of the areola can enlarge as well. When these changes occur, women often seek to rejuvenate their breasts with a breast lift or "mastopexy" in order to remove the excess skin, tighten and raise the breasts, and reduce the diameter of the areolas. However, it is important to understand that a mastopexy will not significantly change the size of your breasts or give upper breast fullness. For women that want smaller, perkier breasts, a breast reduction is recommended. If a woman wants upper breast fullness and/or larger breasts, then they should consider a breast augmentation along with the mastopexy.

There are three basic types of mastopexies with varying degrees of lifting and scarring. The basic thought is that the more you lift and tighten the breast, the more skin that needs to be removed and therefore more scar that is created. The first is called a "peri-areolar" or "donut" mastopexy. This is really a nipple shifting operation and does not significantly raise the breast. This is performed by first removing a "donut" shaped piece of skin around the areola. Then a deep "purse string" suture is placed and tightened in order to decrease the diameter of the opening and lift the nipple to a higher position. Initially, there will be a small amount of wrinkling around the areola due to the bunching up of the skin, but this tends to resolve completely within 3-6 months after surgery. The second type of mastopexy is also called a "lollipop lift" due to the shape of the scar. There will be a round scar around the areola plus a vertical scar extending down to the level of the breast fold (where the lower part of the breast meets the chest). By removing some vertical lower breast skin, the breasts and nipples will both be lifted. The third type of lift is the "anchor" mastopexy. In addition to the lollipop shaped scar, a horizontal scar is added along the breast fold in order to remove large quantities of skin and give the maximum lift.

Women who have asymmetries in nipple height, nipples that point downward, nipples that are below the breast fold, large areolas, elongated breasts, or uneven breasts are typically good candidates for a breast lift.

Frequently Asked Questions About Breast Lifts/Mastopexy

Will a mastopexy change my nipple sensation?

Depending on which type of mastopexy you undergo, there is some risk to losing nipple sensation. The "donut" lift has minimal risk, while the "anchor" lift has the highest risk. All of the lifts are designed to try to preserve the tissue that normally contains the nerves that lead to the nipple. However, there are many anatomic variants relating to where the nerves travel. Nerves that do not follow the "normal" course within your breasts may be damaged to the point of permanent numbness. Most patients experience at least a temporary change in nipple sensation due to stretching and repositioning of the nerves. Most women recover full sensation within 3-12 months after surgery. A small percentage of women never regain normal sensation.

Can I have breast implants placed the same day as my mastopexy?

Yes, it's possible to insert breast implants the day of the mastopexy as long as the size is not excessive. I prefer to do the lift first and then add the implants through a separate site (such as the underarm). That way, we can see exactly how large an implant can be safely placed without putting undue tension on the repair. Also, if a woman has asymmetric breasts, putting the implants in after the lift allows better volume control to achieve better symmetry. If a patient wants a breast lift and very large implants, then I usually recommend that we do the breast lift first and add the implants approximately two months later.

Will I be able to breast-feed if I have a breast lift?

Mastopexy involves removing excess skin from the breast and does not divide the milk ducts so breast function is preserved. Some women experience a tight feeling with breast engorgement after breast lifting which will make breast-feeding more uncomfortable. Also, pregnancy can ruin the results of the breast lift. Therefore, except in cases of unacceptable drooping or asymmetry, I typically recommend that mastopexies be performed once a woman is reasonably sure she is finished with childbearing.

CHAPTER 9

Breast Reduction

Some women have large, disproportionate breasts for their frame size and large breasts frequently cause neck and back pain. They also may have a negative affect on an active lifestyle. A breast reduction procedure can relieve the back and neck pain, regain a youthful appearance and let the patient return to a more active lifestyle.

Some women just want a relatively small breast reduction and if they have nice, relatively perky breasts to begin with, then we can perform liposuction on the breasts and take them down about a cup size, possibly a cup size and a half. This is a relatively simple procedure.

If the patient has breasts with a sagging, unattractive shape, and the nipples are pointing downward, they will not be a good candidate for breast liposuction. In that case we would have to remove some of the excessive skin along with the tissue of the breast and shift the nipple up to a higher position in order to have an aesthetically pleasing breast when we're finished. In an ideal breast, the nipple is going to point horizontal and the nipple also is going to be fairly close to center or just slightly below center on the breast mound itself.

To remove that skin and shift the nipple up, there is going to be some scarring. Typically there will be a "lollipop" shaped scar where there will be a scar around the areola and then a vertical scar going down the breast. In some patients if we have to take out more skin, there will be an "anchor" shaped scar on the breast. The scarring can be similar to what one would experience with a breast lift.

Although some surgeons will actually take the nipple off and then put it back on at the end as a free graft, I've always designed the operation to shift the nipple without removal. If the nipple is taken off and put back, the blood flow to the nipple and the sensation will be gone. I've always performed the operation to preserve the blood flow and the sensation to the nipple.

We have never lost a blood flow, but about 1% or 2% of the time women lose the sensation during a breast reduction and that's generally because the nerves are not always where they're supposed to be. Just the same as we're different anatomically on the outside, sometimes on the inside, the nerves are not at their correct location and they can get damaged during the surgery. Ninety-eight-plus percent of women retain sensation after breast reduction.

CHAPTER 10

Mommy Makeover

Being a mother and experiencing your children growing up is one of the greatest joys in life for a woman. At the same time there are many physical changes to a woman's body after pregnancy, especially if she had multiple births. The physical changes can often be recognized from the face down to the thighs.

After breast-feeding, the breasts can lose volume and projection. They may drop and change shape and sometimes they are not symmetric. The skin in the abdomen stretches during pregnancy beyond its ability to repair itself, so stretch marks are likely to appear. When a mother starts losing weight after childbirth, the skin in her abdomen becomes loose.

When a woman is pregnant, hormones are given off to weaken connective tissues so that the baby can pass through the birth canal. This causes the rectus muscle (the vertical "the six-pack") to move apart and results in ballooning of the abdomen. Hormones also tend to cause fat to be attached to some areas where there wasn't much fat before.

"Saddlebags" may develop in the outer thighs and we frequently see more fat in the flanks, or "love handles" at the waist.

After having children the mother's figure is different than before. A good diet and exercise regimen helps lose much of the fat, but no matter how hard she tries, the shape is not changing back to what it was before having children. The goal of a "mommy makeover" is to try and reestablish what a mother looked like before she was pregnant. In some cases, we can even make them look better than they looked before.

The motivation to have a mommy makeover often comes when a mother looks in the mirror and decides she wants to get some of her youthfulness back. The children are generally now in school and she wants to do something for herself so she can look good in a swimsuit or in tight fitting clothes again.

Every mother's figure is unique and there is not one set of procedures that are prescribed for a "mommy makeover." Some women are interested in improving the appearance of their breasts, while others want to get back a trimmer figure around the mid-section, thighs, or hips. Some are interested in a complete makeover, with changes to the breasts as well as abdomen and thighs.

We frequently perform a breast lift or mastopexy when the nipples are pointing down or are hanging too low. We can usually perform the mastopexy using an incision around the areola or nipple so the resulting scar will not be obvious. If the breasts have lost their volume or projection we often use implants to restore the beauty and give the breasts a plump, youthful look. If the patient needs both a breast lift and implants, we typically combine the surgeries in the same day. To learn more about breast lifts and implants, please refer to Chapters 7 and 8.

A tummy tuck, or abdominoplasty is commonly performed as part of a mommy makeover. With this procedure we can tighten up the rectus muscle, flattening the abdomen and removing loose stretched skin. We may also use liposuction to remove excess fat in the abdomen, love handles, back, or thighs. We typically perform the liposuction and a tummy tuck, if indicated, in the same surgery. More information on liposuction and tummy tucks can be found in Chapter 6. We can also use a laser to make stretch marks less noticeable.

Frequently Asked Questions About a Mommy Makeover

When should I consider a mommy makeover?

Since each pregnancy can affect the figure, a mother should be pretty sure that she is finished with childbearing before having a mommy makeover. When you have decided that you want to get your youthful appearance back and look good again in a two-piece swimsuit or tight fitting clothes, the time may be right for you. Most often, women interested in a mommy makeover are in their thirties or forties.

We like to be sure before we do a tummy tuck that a woman is finished having children for a couple reasons. First, if she had another child she would, of course, ruin the tummy tuck. But more importantly, because we tighten the muscles in most cases, if she got pregnant again, the tight muscles might restrict the baby's growth and there have been reports of higher miscarriage rates in women that have had tummy tucks.

If I am interested in having work done on the breasts and also a tummy tuck and liposuction, can all of these be done at the same time?

Most of the time we can do it all together, even if they need implants, a breast lift, lipo, and a tummy tuck. These procedures can typically all be done in the same day. If the surgery gets to be six hours or longer, we typically keep the patient overnight in our overnight facility. If we do the surgery at the hospital, we keep the patient overnight at the hospital. With a combination of all of these procedures there will be a lot of anesthesia and we want to be able to be sure we manage their pain well, especially on the night of surgery. We want the patient walking around because the best way to prevent any blood clots is to walk around. If they were to go home, chances are they wouldn't be motivated to walk around, but with the nurses here, they will definitely walk them around.

When you do surgery in multiple body areas, all those areas are going to swell up a little bit. That water's got to come from somewhere to get sucked out of the blood vessels.

If the person went home, chances are they could not drink enough water to keep up with that swelling that's going on, and the kidneys would not see enough water for the first day or so, and that's a bad situation. If they stay overnight, then they can have an IV going and the kidneys stay flushed and happy, and everything works out much better.

If for some reason I divide up the breast and the abdominal work at a different time, how long between surgeries should I wait?

I recommend typically at least 6 weeks between the first surgery and the next one, just to make sure everything is well healed and the body has had a chance to recover before having another major operation.

Patient History: 34 Year old mother of 4 who underwent liposuction and tummy tuck. After photos are 3 months post-op.

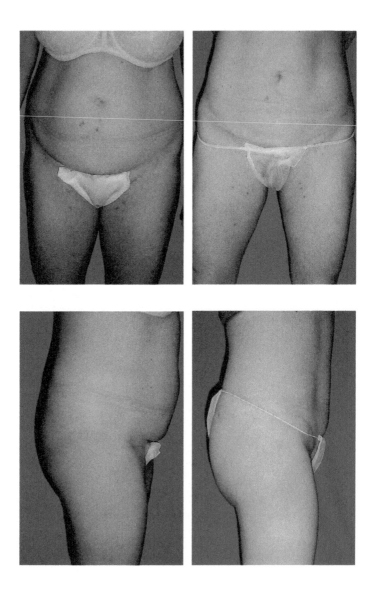

CHAPTER 11

Weight Loss Makeover

I see many patients that have lost a significant amount of weight, 50 pounds to over 100 pounds. This is generally after bariatric surgery with a gastric bypass, lap band, or gastric sleeve. It's really fantastic. They look a lot better in clothes. But they have a lot of loose skin and you can't possibly exercise enough to lose the loose skin.

The loose skin can be from the neck to the knees. I see people, even in their thirties, that have a lot of hanging skin on the neck, like a "waddle." We would address this with a facelift procedure. Another bothersome area with major weight loss is in the arms, especially the upper arms. They can have hanging skin like an "angel wing" when the arms are extended. That skin has limited ability to shrink back because of stretch marks or it's just loose skin. It's difficult to hide, so they don't want to wear a short sleeve shirt. Often the breasts have fallen and there is loose skin all around the waist area. The thighs often have loose skin as well, so they don't look good in shorts and often the buttocks droops.

We have procedures to transform all of these areas and help you realize the beautiful new shape that may be hidden beneath the excess skin that remains, even after you have achieved your goal weight. The first thing we would do during a consult with patients is try to assess their motivation, what they hope to gain from having the surgery and their priority in terms of what they want done first. If they don't have a particular priority, I would typically recommend that we start with the abdominal area.

We want to make sure the weight is stabilized for at least six months before we do the surgery. If the patient is still losing weight, the body is in somewhat of a weakened state, which is not a good time to have surgery. We also do extensive blood work to make sure their nutritional status is good. Often, after having gastric bypass, part of the intestine is bypassed, and there can be some significant vitamin shortages. There can be low levels of protein in their body, and that would indicate a higher risk of wound-healing problems or a slow recovery. We want to make sure that the patient is optimized before they have surgery. I suggest readers review Chapter 13 on nutritional supplements for a healthy body.

I generally perform a "circumferential lower body lift," also known as a "circumferential tuck" or "extended tummy tuck" to remove the excess skin in the abdomen and all around the waist. Sometimes this procedure is combined with liposuction to achieve a beautiful sculpted shape again. At the same time we can lift the outer thighs and lift the buttocks as well. The lower body lift requires an incision all around the circumference of the body, so there will be a scar; however, I always have the patient bring a swimsuit or wear underwear that approximates the dimensions of a swimsuit so we can conceal the scarring in the area that will be covered by the swimsuit.

After the abdominal surgery is performed, patients typically go on to lose some additional weight. This may cause some additional sagging in the breasts, so I generally recommend not to have a breast lift until about two months after the abdominal work to see if there has been additional weight loss that will affect the breasts. It's the breasts that have the highest chance of losing a good result if they lose weight after the surgery. If they had the breast procedure first and then lost weight, the breasts would tend to sag again, and then the patient might need to come back and have a second breast lift. Depending on the look the patient is trying to achieve, we may also combine augmentation with a breast lift.

The skin on the arms can also be removed either by itself as a standalone procedure or in combination with other procedures on the same day. There would typically be a scar from the elbows down to the underarm area, and the scar can be either in the groove between the biceps and the triceps muscles on the front of the arm, or we can put the scar on the back of the arm, pretty much in the triceps area, depending on where the patient prefers the scar to be. Liposuction is sometimes used as well to remove fat and sculpt the arms.

We generally address the outer thighs during the circumferential lower body lift. For many patients we need to address the inner thighs as well. There are two ways to lift the inner thighs. Depending on where they have the looseness will determine which procedure we perform. There's a horizontal thigh lift where the skin is removed from the inner thigh and the scar ends up in the groin, and that scar can be hidden in a swimsuit. If the loose skin is all the way down to the knees, then we do a vertical side tuck, in which skin is removed on the inner aspect of the thigh from the knee all the way up to the groin. There will be a scar there as well, but the only way to get the leg tight and firm is to take skin from the knee all the way up to the groin area. We commonly combine this procedure with liposuction to remove unwanted fat and to sculpt the leg.

Readers interested in knowing more about these procedures are advised to read Chapter 6 on body contouring, Chapter 7 on breast augmentation and Chapter 8 on breast lifts.

Patient History: 36 year old female who underwent liposuction of the abdomen, back, and flanks along with a circumferential lower body lift. After photos are 3 months post-op.

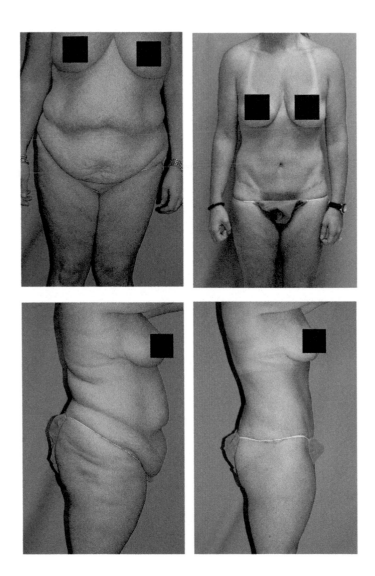

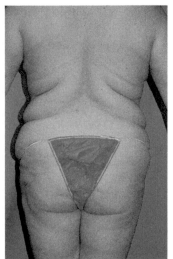 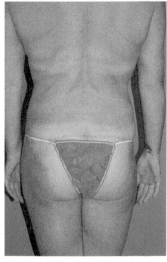

CHAPTER 12

Procedures for Men

Traditionally the vast majority of plastic surgery patients have been women, but men are increasing becoming interested in improving their appearance. Preference for certain procedures depends on the age. A lot of men, as they get older and they have to compete with a younger workforce, come in for facial rejuvenation. They feel like they don't interview as well when they're competing with younger guys for the same job. If they're equally qualified, they believe the younger person would probably get the position. Signs of facial aging often appear in the eyelids. The upper eyelids tend to droop as we age and the lower eyelids develop puffy bags. Eyelid surgery is designed to remove the accumulated fat deposits from the upper and lower eyelids. The result is a facial appearance that makes the patient look years younger.

Flat cheeks are another typical sign of aging. As we age, the facial fat atrophies and thins out, and the face starts to sag and fall and the cheeks flatten. We can easily plump up those areas with injectable fillers and do it slowly and gradually, so that no one even notices they're having it done. It's not a sudden thing where one day they look totally different than they did the day before. Men, in general, appreciate the slow, gradual approach. Botox injections are another common cosmetic procedure for men to decrease wrinkles on the face, making them look younger.

Men are also becoming interested in body contouring. The most common contouring procedure for men is liposuction, especially of the abdomen and flanks. Guys tend to pack their weight around their midsection, whereas for women it's usually more in the thighs. We also occasionally perform tummy tucks on men, particularly when they have lost a lot of weight from diet, exercise or some form of bariatric surgery.

CHAPTER 13

Nutritional Supplements for a Healthy, Attractive Body

A healthy body is more likely to be an attractive body and an unhealthy body is likely going to be less beautiful. Modern farming methods have depleted the soil of vitamins, minerals, and other essential nutrients. I read one study where it was estimated that 97% of Americans are malnourished in some vitamin or mineral. Anyone who wants to stay healthy, improve their immune system, and recover more quickly from illness or surgery should take supplements.

So how can you know which ones to take? Here are some general guidelines:

1) With supplements, you typically get what you pay for. If you buy inexpensive vitamins, then you're probably getting synthetic products that are not well absorbed or utilized by the body.

2) Try to get supplements that come from natural plant sources. These are better utilized by the body. If you

purchase at a natural food store, you are more likely to get high quality products.

3) If you can find the products in capsules or liquid form, then they are easier for your body to digest them when compared to pills.

4) Highly purified products are the best. For example, cheap fish oil can be harmful because it may contain heavy metals like mercury.

5) Pay no attentions to the RDA ("Recommended Daily Allowance") set by the government. This is the minimum you need to stay alive, not to be healthy.

Here is the "Basic Starter Kit" we recommend:

1) A good MULTIVITAMIN + MULTIMINERAL that comes from plant sources.

2) VITAMIN C (take the Ester-C formulation because it is better tolerated by the intestines). Take 500-1,000mg two to three times per day.

3) VITAMIN D3. Ideally, you would have your blood level checked, but most people are deficient because of limited sun exposure. If you are severely deficient, then doctors prescribe 55,000 I.U. per week. For most people, 1,000-5,000 I.U. per day is a good dose. (If everyone followed this one piece of advice, half the cancer doctors would be looking for work 20 years from now.)

4) VITAMIN E (d-alpha tocopherol). This is a fat-soluble vitamin found in nuts, seeds, vegetable oils

and fish oil. It is often found in your multivitamin in sufficient doses.

5) FISH OIL OR KRILL OIL (distilled or pharmaceutical grade purity). Fish oils have many benefits, especially for those with high cholesterol and at risk for heart attack or stroke. (Note: cheap fish oil may have heavy metals like mercury.)

Additional supplements to consider are:

1) COENZYME Q10. This antioxidant is critical for muscle function and energy production. Anyone on statin drugs to lower their cholesterol needs to be on CoQ10 because these drugs lower the CoQ10 levels in your body.

2) ALPHA LIPOIC ACID. A powerful antioxidant that helps maintain optimal blood sugar levels and reduces chance of metabolic syndrome.

3) CURCUMIN. This comes from the spice "turmeric" and has powerful antioxidant and anti-cancer properties.

4) PROBIOTICS. Most meats, that are not organically grown, will have antibiotics in them. These antibiotics will upset the normal bacteria in your colon, which will lower your immune system and deplete you of energy. Taking probiotics (such as Lactobacillus or Acidophilus) will restore your normal intestinal germs. Eating yogurt may also help.

5) TMG (TriMethylGlycine). This reduces high homocysteine levels. High homocysteine levels have

been strongly linked to heart attack and stroke. If fact, checking your homocysteine levels is even more important than having your cholesterol checked.

6) MELATONIN and/or TRYPTOPHAN. Melatonin is an antioxidant that's produced when we sleep. As we age, we produce less melatonin; as a result, our sleep patterns are not as restful and it makes us more prone to illness and rapid aging.

7) DHEA. This is the master hormone of the body and other hormones are created as this large molecule breaks down. As we age, we produce less DHEA and start noticing obvious signs of aging. Even though this can be purchased as an over-the-counter supplement, I strongly recommend you have your blood levels of DHEA checked and have a physician knowledgeable in DHEA follow you.

8) ASTAXANTHIN. This is an antioxidant 40 times more powerful than Vitamin E.

CHAPTER 14

Skin Care and Slowing Down the Aging Process

Having beautiful skin is one of the most obvious hallmarks of health and youthfulness. Taking good care of your skin will not only make you look better, it may prevent skin cancer. It's never too early to start taking care of your skin. Sunscreen, protective clothing, and hats should be used in childhood. People should consider medical grade skin care even in their 20s or 30s. If you're older than that, go ahead and start now. Your skin will not only look better, but it will heal faster if you have any resurfacing procedures or surgery.

Your skin is a marvelous organ made up of two distinct layers: the epidermis (superficial) and dermis (deep). The superficial part of the epidermis is composed of a protective layer of dead keratinocytes. The deep layer of the epidermis has living cells such as melanocytes which release melanin to give the skin a tan or brown pigment. The dermis is much thicker than the epidermis and all of it is composed of living cells. You will also find complex structures such as oil glands, sweat glands, and hair follicles either in the dermis or just deep into it. Coursing throughout the dermis, there is an interwoven net of collagen and elastin fibers which hold everything together and give skin its' pliable nature. The collagen keeps your skin from stretching too far and the elastin fibers allow the skin to snap back after being stretched.

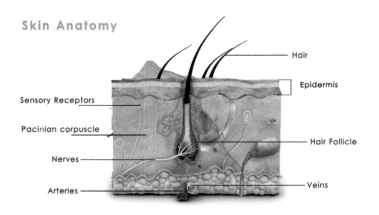

Skin Anatomy

Youthful skin has a thin epidermis and thick dermis. As we age, the epidermis gets thicker and the dermis gets thinner. As a result, the skin starts to look dull and loses its' elasticity. Wrinkles soon follow. Splotchy pigmentation also occurs; especially those who have had extensive sun exposure. The skin can become flakey in areas, which may indicate pre-cancerous or even cancerous lesions.

If you are considering a facelift, then you should definitely invest in skin care as well. Without proper skin care, you won't get as good a result from your facelift, nor will it last as long. The rejuvenation process will be woefully incomplete. With proper skin care, your skin will be thicker, more elastic, have more even pigment, and a healthier color…all the signs of youth.

You may have heard the terms "free radicals" and "antioxidants" in the past and wondered how that relates to you and to the aging process. When you hear the term "free radical," you might be thinking of someone with extreme views who wreaks havoc to bring about drastic political, economic, or social reform. However, this is not what we are going to talk about. Free radicals are simply atoms or molecules with an unpaired electron. This makes the atom or molecule unstable. These free radicals then go around wreaking havoc by stealing electrons from other molecules to satisfy their need for stability by having a complete set of electrons. A chain reaction like falling dominoes then occurs because new free radicals are formed which then go about stealing electrons from other molecules. Free radicals are everywhere! They are in the air we breathe, in our bodies, in your car that is starting to slowly rust, in the plastic that's drying out and changing color, in the wall paint that's fading…you get the point. In our bodies, we create free radicals just by breathing or breaking down food to give off energy. When oxygen breaks down to release energy, oxygen free radicals are formed which lead to "oxidative stress." So, free radicals have a useful purpose in that they allow energy production. However, the oxidative stress that follows can be very dangerous in that it leads to cell damage at the level of the DNA and mitochondria (which are like little energy factories inside each cell). As this damage accumulates over time, cells become weaker. Weak cells are not only responsible for the signs of aging, they also lead to age related diseases such as dementia, Alzheimer's, cancer, arthritis, atherosclerosis, and diabetes.

Fortunately, our marvelous bodies produce little brave champions called "antioxidants" to rid ourselves of these little scavengers. Antioxidants are "unselfish" molecules that gladly give up an electron to a free radical and yet at the same time remain stable themselves. This neutralizes the free radical and makes it harmless. There are many enzyme systems in the body that produce antioxidants, but the primary antioxidants that we need to get from dietary intake are Vitamin C (ascorbic acid), Vitamin E (d-alpha tocopherol), Beta carotene (which is transformed into Vitamin A in our bodies) and flavonoids. Vitamin C is water soluble and is commonly found in citrus fruits, kiwi, berries, and brightly colored veggies such as red peppers, broccoli, kale, and spinach. Vitamin E is fat soluble and is present in nuts, seeds, vegetal and fish oils, whole grains, and apricots. Beta carotene is a precursor to Vitamin A (retinol) and is found in liver, egg yolk, milk, butter, spinach, carrots, squash, broccoli, yams, tomatoes, grains, and certain fruits such as cantaloupe and peaches. Eating five daily servings of organic fruits or vegetables should provide you with enough antioxidants to be healthy. Be sure to vary your fruits and vegetables as well so you don't eat the same things every day. Athletes may need more antioxidants and often take oral supplements to protect their bodies from the additional oxidative stress produced during vigorous exercise.

Environmental factors can also increase free radical damage. The top culprits are excessive sun exposure, smoking, and pollutants in the air, food, and water. All these factors lead to DNA damage as well as destruction of the collagen and elastin fibers in your skin. This causes the skin to thin out, lose elasticity, and form wrinkles. So, in addition to proper dietary intake of fruits and vegetables, what else can you do to slow down the aging process? Follow the guidelines below and you'll not only improve your skin, you'll improve your overall health as well.

I'm going to give you a huge money-saving tip: don't waste your money on skin care products you can buy at a mall or online. I don't care if it costs $400 for a little jar of the product; it won't help slow your skin's aging process. Even if they have some of the same ingredients found in prescription strength products, these products will be too weak to cause effective long-term changes in the skin. In addition, they are likely to be in the wrong combination with other ingredients or not have the proper carrier molecules to drive these ingredients deep into your skin where they can do the most good. Over the counter skin care products cannot change the structure of the skin or else they would be classified as "prescription" by the FDA. The most you can hope for is a temporary improvement in your skin. Typically, the results fade within a few days of stopping these products.

On the other hand, prescription-strength skin care products will go deep into the skin to change the actual structure of skin. For example, new elastic collagen can form, age spots can be eliminated, wrinkles can soften, redness (such as rosacea) can resolve, and a whole host of other skin disorders can be resolved. Amazingly, despite the far superior benefits, the cost of these prescription-strength products is usually comparable to the less-effective over-the-counter products.

In this brief discussion, I cannot possibly give you exact advice that will guarantee great skin results. Your skin is unique and will need a certified skin care expert to guide you through this process. Though we make the best guess at what will work for you, some of this will be trial and error. Eventually, your skin can look gorgeous, but don't expect instant results. Any skin care regimen will typically take at least 2-3 months before you begin to notice a significant change. That's because the deepest layers of skin take about a month before they reach the surface and slough off.

Tips for Beautiful Skin and Slowing Down the Aging Process

1) Avoid excessive sun exposure or tanning beds. Please notice I said "excessive." Limited sun exposure is considered healthy in moderate doses. It not only allows your skin to produce Vitamin D, it also helps with mood. Burning your skin is never good and indicates irreversible damage to your skin structures. Ultraviolet

rays are constantly causing damage to the deep layers of skin as well. This causes the classic signs, such as loss of elasticity, wrinkles, saggy skin, splotchy pigment, dark lesions, scaly growths, and even skin cancer. Use a good sunblock with an SPF of 30 or higher that covers both UVA and UVB rays if you're going to be out in the sun more than 15 minutes. The best sunscreens have titanium or zinc because they physically block the ultraviolet rays. If you're going to be in direct sun or getting wet or sweaty, reapply the sunscreen every two hours. If you're not willing to protect your skin from ongoing damage, then it's probably best not to even bother with a skin care regimen.

2) Smoking is one of the worse things you can do for your skin and overall health. Smoking or ingesting second-hand smoke has clearly been shown to not only lead to increased rates of various forms of cancer and lung disease, but also to damaged skin. Not only is there a toxic chemical assault on your body, the nicotine in cigarettes also has been shown to shrink small blood vessels which feed the skin. If skin has poor blood flow, it will age faster. Studies of identical twins, in which only one of the twins smoked, showed startling differences in their appearance. The middle-aged smoker twin typically looked 10-20 years older than the non-smoker.

3) If possible, don't live in the center of a city. Studies have shown that if you stand at the street corner of a

busy city, you will inhale more pollutants in 10 minutes than our ancestors encountered in an entire lifetime.

4) Buy only organic food. Non-organic food is typically genetically modified so it can tolerate higher levels of pesticides and herbicides therefore leading to a higher yield of a crop.

5) Avoid sugar, grains, processed foods, and trans fats (also called partially hydrogenated oils). I'm sure you've seen the government's food pyramid that shows grains, bread, and pasta at the bottom and protein and fat at the top. Think about it. This is how Americans have been taught to eat for over 50 years. Where has it gotten us? We're the fattest people on the planet. The government food pyramid is the # 1 cause of obesity and obesity-related illness in this country. The food pyramid has nothing to do with your health. It was just a way for the government to support the American farmer. There is not a nutritionist in the world that will tell you that this is a healthy way to live. You need much more protein and fat (yes, I said fat) in your diet if you want to be healthy. Sugar and grains will cause a spike in your blood sugar. Your pancreas will give off insulin to lower your blood sugar. Where does that sugar go? Some of it will go to your liver; some to your muscles; but the majority will end up in your fat cells. If you have a low fat diet, the body will want more calories for energy and you will overeat in the form of carbohydrates. Processed foods and trans fats contain ingredients that are toxic and

lead to weight gain, heart disease, diabetes, dementia, and a whole host of other problems. Taking in healthy omega 3 fats such as pure fish oil, krill oil, or olive oil will also help your skin to be more supple. Take the time to educate yourself on proper diet and you will enjoy a happier, more energetic, and disease-free life.

6) Drink plenty of water. Water is essential to life and all the thousands of chemical processes that occur in your body every day. There's a lot of controversy as to how much water you should drink. There are advocates that say, "just drink when you're thirsty." The problem with that mentality is that the body will adjust to just about any lifestyle you give it. In other words, if you are not in the habit of drinking much water, then your body will accommodate to that amount of water as its set point. Also, as we age, the thirst mechanisms changes and we feel less thirsty. Many elderly people walk around chronically dehydrated. This can lead to fatigue, light-headedness, constipation, dry skin, headaches, excessive hunger, and a whole host of other problems. So just how much water is enough? First, let me say that I recommend you buy a good filtration system for your water. Municipal water is a wonderful thing, but it can contain toxic chlorine, fluoride, traces of multiple medications, heavy metals, and many other impurities. Second, put some water in a glass (not plastic) container and try to leave it in the refrigerator at least several hours before drinking it. This will allow some of the residual chlorine to escape the water. Third, drink as

much water as you need so that your urine will be a very, very pale yellow color. Fourth, drink 1-2 glasses of water as soon as you get up before having breakfast to allow your body to flush out the impurities it has mobilized while you slept.

7) Exercise your body regularly. Try to do aerobic exercise and some strength training 3-5 times per week. Without exercise, your muscles will atrophy at an alarming rate due to loss of proper hormone balance (see below). Check with your doctor before starting any vigorous training regimen. There are hundreds of studies that show that exercise fights the loss of stamina, muscle strength, balance, and bone density that increases with age. If you need help with understanding what exercises are worth doing, ask a knowledgeable friend or hire a fitness coach.

8) Get plenty of sleep. Your body and brain repair themselves when you sleep. Without at least 6 hours of sleep, you will age faster and have increased risks of depression, heart attack, stroke, unfavorable mood, fatigue, bouts of anger, viral sickness, and mental deterioration (such as dementia). So, aim for 8 hours of sleep to improve your mood, physical health, and longevity.

9) Exercise your brain regularly. This can be done in an infinite number of ways. You can read, do crossword puzzles, learn a new language, write letters, build something with your hands, paint or draw pictures, or

get online to the many websites that are designed to stimulate brain health.

10) Fast intermittently. Fasting allows your body to naturally detoxify and cleanse itself. You could start by fasting for 12-16 hours once a week. This could be as easy as skipping breakfast. After a few weeks, you can increase it to a 24 hour fast. Eventually, you may be able to increase it to two days. If you are over 40 or have any significant medical problems, be sure to consult with your doctor before fasting over 24 hours.

11) Develop your spirit. Many studies have shown that religion and spirituality have many positive physical and emotional benefits. In addition, research on prayer, meditation, and learning to forgive has clear benefits in terms of happiness as well as social interactions.

12) Consider hormone replacement therapy. Some scientists consider this the number 1 weapon against the signs and symptoms of aging. As we age, cumulative cell damage eventually leads to diminished or improper hormone production. Hormones are little chemical messengers that tell other cells or organs what to do. If those hormones are out of whack, you are not going to feel good. The typical signs are loss of energy, libido (sex drive), and stamina. You may also experience weight gain or fat accumulations in areas that never bothered you before. Your muscles begin to atrophy. Weight loss also becomes increasingly difficult. As if that wasn't enough, your skin becomes thinner

and starts to wrinkle. Hormones start to diminish at around the age of 35. I would strongly encourage you to only go to a physician that prescribes bio-identical hormones. Other patented hormone treatments (typically put out by drug companies) can have serious side effects, such as cancer. These hormones may help with your symptoms, but they are not identical to what your body would normally produce. Bio-identical hormones are by far the best because your body will react properly to them. For more in depth information, I would recommend you read any of Suzanne Somers' books on this subject. They provide extensive, easy to understand information from the world's experts in the field.

13) Take vitamins and antioxidant supplements. I am often asked if nutritional supplements are really necessary. Can't you get enough nutrients by eating healthy? The answer is yes, but needs to be qualified. If you were to eat 5-6 servings daily of organic fruits and vegetables and avoided all processed foods, you would be reasonably healthy. However, if you want to give your body all the essential nutrients you need to combat disease and aging, you would have to eat 5,000 to 6,000 calories per day. Unless you were a top athlete who could burn off this many calories per day, you would gain 2-3 pounds per week (which is hardly considered healthy). So, for optimum health, vitality, disease prevention, and longevity, I would highly recommend you take high

quality nutritional supplements. See Chapter 13 for recommended nutritional supplements.

14) Dry skin is thinner than well-hydrated skin and therefore wrinkles more easily and looks less healthy. Be sure to hydrate well and take in essential fats before purchasing moisturizers. Moisturizers contain water and lipids (fats) which will temporarily plump up the skin and make it appear more youthful.

15) As mentioned above, antioxidants are important for overall health. However, you probably can't consume enough antioxidants to make a significant impact on your skin. Fortunately, there are topical products which contain antioxidants such as Vitamin C and E which can greatly aid in rejuvenating the skin.

16) Retinols are one of the active forms of Vitamin A. When you ingest foods such as liver, eggs, dark veggies, cheese, or milk, your body has to convert the "provitaimin" into the active vitamin. Vitamin A is essential for good vision (especially night vision), bone health, immune function, and healthy skin. Topical retinols have been around for many years and there have been numerous scientific studies proving their benefits. Many over-the-counter products tout "retinol" as one of their ingredients. However, these products have such a small amount of retinol that it does not reach the threshold for effectiveness. Retinol (Retin-A, tretinoin, Renova, etc) causes increased turnover of cells in the skin. Both the superficial layer

(epidermis) and deep layer (dermis) thicken due to new collagen formation and increased blood flow. It also causes a more uniform pigmentation to the skin. Unfortunately, many patients experience irritation, redness, discomfort and scaliness soon after beginning treatment. All these symptoms are normal and if you continue to use the Retinol, you will eventually stop having these symptoms and begin to enjoy the benefits of the product. Your dose or frequency may need to be adjusted, so be sure to ask your skin care expert for details.

17) When the melanin-producing cells get overstimulated (either from excessive sun exposure, burns, chronic irritation, etc), splotchy tan or brown spots can appear on the skin. Topical agents such as hydroquinone, azaleic acid, or kojic acid can all help minimize these spots. Hydroquinone in a 4% strength is the most commonly used agent. Again, beware of over-the-counter products containing hydroquinone in weaker formulations that are essentially ineffective.

CHAPTER 15

Tips for a Faster Recovery

There are a number of things patients can do to speed up their recovery. Your plastic surgeon will provide a set of post-operative instructions that include showering, dressing changes and other things that need to be done. Following the post-operative instructions makes a large difference. Light exercise like walking is generally recommended. Eating healthy foods, including lean proteins such as chicken or fish after surgery will help you heal faster. We also recommend avoiding excessive carbohydrates after surgery as they actually hinder healing.

Patients that are well nourished are going to heal faster than those that have vitamin or mineral deficiencies. Nutrition also influences the body's ability to make a good scar that will be less visible over time. A scar itself is mainly collagen and does not have built-in oil glands like other skin. You need the right nutritional building blocks to develop good collagen and if you have good collagen you will develop a better scar. For this reason we encourage all of our patients to take vitamins and minerals ahead of their surgeries and we give all of our patients nutritional supplements that we recommend for quicker recovery. In addition to multivitamins, extra vitamin C can help build collagen faster and help the tissues heal faster. Extra vitamin D can help people resist infection more and strengthen their immune systems, leading to a faster recovery. See the information provided in Chapter 13 for more information on recommended nutritional supplements.

Patients should ask their plastic surgeon for advice on scar care after surgery. Proper topical treatment of the scar after surgery with scar care products or covering with a special tape is very important. On a microscopic level, the scar can crack and bacteria can fall into the cracks and cause inflammation, which leads to a thicker scar. Patients that take good care of their scars will end up with a thinner and paler scar.

There are certain genetic predispositions to making an attractive scar. Some people make very thick scars that are called keloids. There's not a lot you can do to change your genetic disposition. Occasionally if a scar starts getting thick, we can inject a little bit of steroid into the scar or we also have a laser that is very useful to help flatten out thicker scars. We usually wait at least one or two months before injecting any steroid or using any laser procedures on the scars.

Scars can also hyper-pigment and that's also typically a genetic predisposition. People that tan very easily or dark-skinned people often will form dark scars. There is a chemical called hydroquinone that can be applied to the scar topically to help lighten that color. Over-the-counter hydroquinone is very ineffective, but prescription strength hydroquinone will significantly lighten the scar within a few months and it will blend in much better.

It's important for patients to know in advance what to do if they are having a problem after surgery. If there's ever a question about the way the healing is going, the best thing to do is always to call the plastic surgeon's office. One of the questions that might be useful in asking ahead of time is if something happens at night, who should the patient call? What phone number should they call and who should they expect will answer the call? Will it be a nurse? Will it be the plastic surgeon? Will it be a cross-covering plastic surgeon? Typically, the call system should be set up that a patient should have a return phone call, at the most, within 15 minutes of them calling with a situation or a problem. Because there are so many possible things, so many questions that could come up, if there's ever a concern in the patient's mind, the safest thing is to always to call the plastic surgeon and find out if the condition is of any concern.

CHAPTER 16

How to Maintain Your Body Contouring Results

After performing over 10,000 body contouring procedures, I have sadly noticed that about 15% of my patients go on to gain weight after surgery and therefore lose much of what they gained by having surgery. This information is provided to help you maintain and hopefully enhance your final body contours. Bad information is typically what has led most people to gain weight so replacing it with good information is the key to empowering you to take control of your physique. Here are some basic dietary and exercise tips that should help you.

Diet

1) **DRINK ONLY WATER.** Many patients think they are being healthy by drinking diet sodas or fruit juice. Nothing could be farther from the truth. Studies show that people that drink diet sodas gain more weight than those that drink sugary sodas. Fruit juices give you

instant elevation of your blood sugar levels. The body must combat this by secreting the hormone "insulin." The insulin will quickly drive that sugar into your fat cells to bring the blood sugar levels back to normal. Therefore, fruit juices also make you fat. So drink just pure water (add lemon or lime juice for flavor if desired). You should drink enough water that your urine is a very pale yellow color.

2) **AVOID OR SEVERELY LIMIT ALCOHOL.** Alcohol has a TRIPLE WHAMMY effect. First, it is a source of empty sugar calories that get stuffed into your fat cells. Second, it causes increased uric acid levels, which put you in "hibernation" or "fat storing" mode. Third, it slows down your metabolism so it's even harder to lose fat. So, the maximum alcohol you should have is 1 or 2 five-ounce drinks per week.

3) **EAT FAT.** One of the myths of dieting is that you should avoid fat. If you do, your body sends off "famine" hormones that cause you to store more calories in the fat cells. Be sure to eat modest amounts of the right fats such as olive oil, fish oil, or coconut oil. Nuts are also a healthy form of fat. Never eat fried foods. Eat grass-fed red meat once a week at most.

4) **SHOP THE PERIPHERY OF THE GROCERY STORE.** In other words, avoid buying processed foods typically found in the center aisles as much as possible. Processed foods have chemicals, which your body will try to shuttle away from your vital organs and stuff it into the (you guessed it) fat cells!

5) **FORGET THE WHITE FOODS; GO FOR COLOR.** This means that "white" foods such as bread, rice, pasta, sugar, potatoes, etc. are what cause weight gain. These foods all have a high "glycemic index" and should be avoided. You should eat multiple helpings of colorful veggies and fruit every day (but not bananas).

6) **EVERY MEAL OR SNACK SHOULD HAVE BALANCED CARBOS, PROTEIN, AND FAT.** If you need detailed instructions on this, please read "The Zone" diet books by Dr. Barry Sears.

7) **CHECK YOUR HORMONES.** If you're still having problems losing weight, see your doctor to have your thyroid, DHEA, and sex hormone (testosterone, estrogen, and progesterone) levels checked. If these are sub-optimal, weight loss is extremely difficult.

Exercise

1) **CHECK WITH YOUR DOCTOR BEFORE STARTING ANY EXERCISE PLAN.**

2) **START WITH RESISTANCE TRAINING.** If you only have 3 hours or less to workout per week, do some resistance training. If you have more than 3 hours per week, add some cardio workouts. Resistance training not only burns calories, it increases your metabolism so you continue to burn calories while you sleep and into the next day. Cardio only burns calories while you are doing the exercises.

3) **CONSIDER HIRING A PERSONAL TRAINER.**

4) **MIX IT UP.** Your body has an incredible ability to adapt to your workouts. You should completely change your workout routine about every 6 weeks.

5) **WORKOUT FOR ONLY ABOUT 45-60 MINUTES.** Working out for over an hour will cause depletion of the glucose (sugar) in your liver, which then causes your body to release a hormone called "cortisol." Cortisol is also given off in times of stress. Cortisol reduces muscle mass (which is the engine that burns fat) and causes your body to age faster. It also leads to weight gain.

6) **CONSIDER HIGH INTENSITY INTERVAL TRAINING (HIIT).** HIIT involves bursts of all out exercise for 60-90 seconds followed by slow exercise for about a minute; then repeat. You can try to do this for 6-8 cycles. HIIT has been shown to greatly increase metabolism and burn fat. You can find many good workouts on the Internet.

CHAPTER 17

Anesthesia for Plastic Surgery

Contributed by Vasiliki "Bess" Collins, MD

Frequently Asked Questions About Anesthesia for Plastic Surgery

Do I really need to have anesthesia? After all, it's only plastic surgery.

"Plastic surgery" is defined as "surgery done to repair, restore, or improve lost, injured, defective, or misshapen body parts." Plastic surgery can be classified as "reconstructive" (to re-establish a normal appearance) or "cosmetic" (in order to beautify existing facial or body areas). Because surgery involves cutting the skin, some form of anesthesia must be provided.

As competent board certified surgical professionals, surgeons and anesthesiologists that are proficient in outpatient surgical care should provide patients with the same standards as those found in the best available hospitals. Plastic surgery patients should expect their safety and comfort to be of utmost concern. Anything less would be both substandard and potentially unsafe.

So what exactly is "anesthesia"?

The term anesthesia comes from the Greek for "loss of sensation." Anesthesia is a reversible state that is induced by medications. It can eliminate pain, remove the memory of the procedure or how it felt, and reduce anxiety.

Anesthesia is made as safe as possible by careful calculation of the required dosages and constant monitoring by anesthesia professionals.

What are my anesthesia options?

The primary ways that anesthesia is administered is with local, regional, monitored anesthesia care, or general anesthetics.

Local only - The surgeon will inject local anesthetic at the surgical site in the skin with this approach. An anesthesiologist will not be present to provide sedation or continuously monitor your condition as with the other techniques.

Regional anesthesia - This technique produces numbness with the injection of local anesthesia around nerves in a region of the body corresponding to the surgical procedure. With regional anesthesia, you will feel no pain, and you may be awake or receive sedation to your comfort level with medications injected by IV.

General anesthesia - This anesthetic choice produces unconsciousness so that you will not feel, see, or hear anything during the surgical procedure. General anesthesia is the administration of anesthetic agents through an intravenous method (IV) or inhaled gases that make a person unconscious and unable to feel pain.

The combination of these anesthetic agents is intended to induce:

- Analgesia - loss of response to pain
- Amnesia - loss of memory of the procedure
- Immobility - loss of motor reflexes
- Unconsciousness
- Relaxation of skeletal muscles

Monitored anesthesia care - With this approach, you usually receive pain medication and sedatives through an intravenous (IV) line from your anesthesiologist or nurse anesthetist. The surgeon will inject local anesthesia into the skin, which will provide additional pain control during and after the procedure. While you are sedated, your anesthesiologist or nurse anesthetist will monitor your vital body functions.

The type of anesthesia you receive depends on a number of factors including the type and length of procedure you are having, your medical history, and the anesthesiologist's and surgeon's preference.

Why Would a Doctor Use Only Local Anesthesia?

If a doctor *only* promotes local anesthesia, ask yourself these questions:

- Is the doctor a board certified plastic surgeon who operates in an accredited operating room and has hospital privileges?
- Is he/she fully experienced in all aesthetic procedures of the face and body?
- Does he/she only offer local anesthesia because an anesthesiologist won't come to an office without an accredited operating room?
- Is it better to have the wrong operation under local anesthesia than the correct one under general anesthesia?

The problem with choosing a specific procedure solely because it can be done under local anesthesia is that your surgeon may not be offering you the correct procedure or the safest path to your desired result. You should ask "Why?"

Sometimes the doctor may not know how to perform the appropriate procedure. For example, a doctor may only do liposuction under local anesthesia, but in reality you need a tummy tuck. They may tell you liposuction under local anesthesia is your "only safe option."

It is important to understand that an increasing number of doctors who aren't plastic surgeons, perform cosmetic surgeries learned at weekend courses taught by other nonplastic surgeons. A knowledgeable, informed patient is actually a safer and more satisfied patient.

An experienced board certified plastic surgeon in conjunction with an experienced board certified anesthesiologist will be able to offer you the safest and most effective procedure and the ideal anesthetic so that you may have the absolute best outcome.

What is twilight anesthesia?

"Twilight anesthesia" is a common term used to describe monitored anesthesia care (see above).

What is the difference between a nurse anesthetist (CRNA) and an anesthesiologist? Does it really matter who administers my anesthesia?

There are significant differences in the training, responsibilities, and experience of an anesthesiologist (who is a *physician*) and nurse anesthetists (who are *nurses*).

An **anesthesiologist** is a physician who has specialized in the practice of anesthesia. This requires completion of at least four years of additional residency training after completing an accredited four years of medical school. This additional training prepares anesthesiologists to handle almost any situation that may arise during and after surgical procedures. In addition, since these are medical doctors, they are able to practice *independently*.

In contrast, **nurse anesthetists** have undergone an additional two years of training in anesthesia after completing nursing school. Nurse anesthetists *can't practice independently* of a physician. In the hospital setting they practice under the supervision of an anesthesiologist. In an outpatient plastic surgery center or office where there is no anesthesiologist, the surgeon who is performing the surgery supervises the nurse anesthetists.

When will I be able to speak to my anesthesia provider?

After your procedure is scheduled with your plastic surgeon all pertinent medical data should be forwarded to your anesthesiologist or nurse anesthetist. Upon reviewing your chart, your anesthesia provider should call you to discuss your medical history and inform you of what to expect from your anesthesia experience.

What questions should I expect from my anesthesia provider?

The conversation you have with your anesthesia provider is vital in establishing clear communication so that you become familiar with what will occur before, during, and after your surgery. Issues addressed should include the following:

- A full medical history of all past health issues
- Current height and weight measurement
- Medication list
- Any allergies to medications, foods, or latex
- Substance use (such as smoking, e-cigs, alcohol, illicit drug use)
- Past surgeries

- Past exposure to anesthesia and any secondary history of problems you or your family members have experienced

Your anesthesia provider will advise you how to prepare for your upcoming surgical procedure, life style choices that will be best in preparation for your surgery, and your day of surgery itinerary.

Is my medical history important?

Discussing your medical history in full detail and disclosing all previous health concerns, conditions or required treatments or therapies with your anesthesia provider may be the most significant way you can contribute to a safe and comfortable surgical experience. Knowledge is power for both you as the patient and your anesthesia provider!

Are there any health conditions that will determine if anesthesia will be safe for me?

Factors that can increase your risk of problems under general anesthesia include heart and lung disease, high blood pressure, sleep apnea, gastric reflux, smoking, illegal drug use, and obesity.

The use of aspirin, certain herbal supplements, and non-steroidal anti-inflammatory drugs (such as Advil, Motrin, Ibuprofen) can interfere with blood clotting and can cause excessive bleeding, changes in blood pressure, and can affect anesthesia drugs. Medications that are indicated for seizures or anxiety and depression should also come under scrutiny.

Can I continue my medicines before surgery?

There are many medicines for conditions such as high blood pressure, heart or lung disease, or diabetes that may need to be continued up to and on the day of surgery. Female hormone replacement or birth control pills may need to be stopped before surgery due to the increased risk of blood clots. All medications should be disclosed to assess the need for possibly stopping them before surgery. This is where communication is vital. You and your anesthesia provider should discuss all medications and the plan for continuing or discontinuing them before your scheduled surgery.

Are there things I can do to make my surgery safer?

Yes. Divulge all heath and medication history to both your surgeon and anesthesia provider. The ideal patient has followed the recommended plan as advised by the anesthesia provider, has had adequate nutrition and hydration in the preceding days, and has complied with the medication recommendations.

Why can't I eat and drink before anesthesia?

An appropriate fasting period prior to procedures performed under anesthesia is essential for patient safety. Your stomach should be empty to avoid stomach contents being aspirated into the airway. When you are going under anesthesia, your body and all its functions are temporarily "put to sleep." Therefore normal reactions, like swallowing are altered. Since you may be unable to control your gag reflex, if you eat something before surgery your stomach contents could regurgitate into your airways causing complications such as pneumonia. In severe cases, this can be fatal. It is recommended that you not eat for at least 8 hours before surgery or drink anything for 4 hours or more before surgery. However, if your anesthesia provider recommends that you continue specific medication, you may take it with a sip of water. Fasting before surgery usually includes chewing gum, candy, mints, chewing tobacco, and all beverages including water.

Do I really need to stop smoking and alcohol use before my surgery?

If you are a smoker, your surgeon and anesthesia provider will advise you to quit smoking as soon as possible. Smokers are more likely to experience surgical complications (such as infection, wound-healing problems, thicker scars, etc.) and breathing complications during and after anesthesia (such as bronchitis or pneumonia). Smokers must also be especially careful to carry out deep breathing exercises after their surgery to prevent chest infection, pneumonia, or other lung problems. An easy to use device called an "incentive spirometer" can be very helpful during recovery from surgery.

Avoiding alcohol intake for at least one week prior to surgery will reduce potential negative effects such as increased bleeding risk, interactions with anesthetic medications, and poor wound healing.

Are herbal supplements, weight loss medications or over the counter medications allowed prior to anesthesia?

Researchers have compiled a list of herbs to avoid in the two weeks prior to surgery and anesthesia:

- For bleeding effects – avoid gingko biloba, garlic, ginseng, dong quai, feverfew, fish oils
- For drug interactions – avoid echinacea, goldenseal, licorice, St. John's wort, kava, valerian root
- For cardiovascular effects – avoid ephedra, garlic
- For anesthetic effects – avoid valerian root, St. John's wort, kava
- For photosensitivity effects – avoid St. John's wort, dong quai
- For hypoglycemia effects – avoid ginseng

As a general rule weight loss supplements should be discontinued at least 2 weeks before surgery.

Over the counter medications like aspirin and other non-steroidal anti-inflammatory drugs (such as Motrin, Ibuprofen, Alleve, etc.) can interfere with blood clotting and should be avoided unless prohibited by your primary care doctor. Cold and allergy preparations will have to be evaluated by the anesthesia provider.

What is my risk for nausea and vomiting after surgery?

There are specific factors that put patients at risk for nausea after surgery. Certain patients, primarily women of childbearing age who are non-smokers, who have a history of motion sickness and are having specific procedures such as gynecological surgery or breast surgery, are more at risk for nausea or vomiting.

Nausea and vomiting after the surgery is not dependent on the length of the anesthetic, but certain types of anesthesia and appropriate preventative drug selection may help to minimize the risk of nausea.

It is important that you disclose to your anesthesia provider any history of motion sickness or previous nausea and vomiting when exposed to anesthesia.

I have a cold or the flu (upper respiratory infection). Will that cause any problems when I receive anesthesia?

Since essentially all cosmetic surgery procedures are elective in nature, the primary goal should be to only operate on and anesthetize those individuals that are at their optimum health. All types of anesthesia may require airway devices. A recent upper respiratory infection can be associated with an irritated airway, increased secretions, and increased oxygen requirements. These issues may actually worsen after an anesthetic.

During anesthesia, an involuntary cough or spasm can constrict the airway and make ventilation, or breathing gas exchange a challenge.

Your anesthesia provider can evaluate any potential problems or concerns about cold or flu symptoms and advise you as to when it would be safe to receive your anesthetic.

Can I have anesthesia without an IV?

In all cases of surgery, one or more intravenous lines are necessary. Frequently, the intravenous is started in the back of the hand, using a small amount of local anesthesia to minimize the discomfort. Other sites can be used as well. The IV is used not only to provide analgesics (pain killers) and anesthetic agents, but also as a route for fluids. The IV also serves as a "lifeline" for the administration of emergency drugs if needed. The IV is removed in the recovery room when there is no further need for intravenous medications.

I am very anxious about my surgery. Can I have something to relax me before I enter the operating room?

It is very natural to be anxious about undergoing a surgical procedure and having to be anesthetized. You should discuss your fears and concerns with your surgeon and anesthesia provider. He or she will be able to help allay your worries. Most anesthesia providers will offer mild sedation after your IV is started. If they do not, you should feel comfortable in requesting medication that will calm you.

What actually happens in the operating room when I have my procedure?

You will enter the operating room and be asked to move to the operating room bed. Your anesthesia provider and nurse will be in total attendance to all your needs. Heart, oxygen, and blood pressure monitors will be placed. You may be asked to breathe pure oxygen for 2-3 minutes through a soft mask. After you are in a deep sleep state induced by medications placed in your IV, airway devices may be placed to insure optimal oxygen delivery.

During surgery you will be monitored very intensively. The advanced medical instruments are used to keep an eye on the function of the heart, lungs, brain and other vital organs, as well as to make sure you are receiving just the right amount of anesthesia. Every patient is an individual and the amount and selection of the proper anesthesia medicines will be the priority of the anesthesia provider. You will be given medications that allow elimination of awareness and pain. When your surgeon finishes your surgery, the anesthesia provider will cease the anesthetics and allow you to awaken comfortably.

I'm afraid I'm going to wake up during my surgery. Is this going to happen?

If you are concerned about this issue, please discuss it with your anesthesia provider before surgery. During general anesthesia, it is extremely rare to experience what is referred to as "recall." However, this is dependent on the anesthetic technique and the amount and type of drugs that are administered by your anesthesiologist or nurse anesthetist. During regional anesthesia (i.e. spinal, epidural, or nerve block) you may choose to be anywhere from wide-awake to fully asleep. Many of the sedatives used have short-term memory-blanking properties, and although you may be awake and conversant during the procedure you may have no recollection of these events later. Your level of consciousness is very much under the control of your anesthesia provider. Your anesthetic can be "customized" to meet your expectations.

What happens after my surgery is over?

After surgery, you will be taken from the operating room to another area, often called the "recovery room," or "post-anesthesia care unit" (PACU). Your anesthesia provider will direct the monitoring and medications needed for your safe recovery. For about the first 30 minutes, specially trained nurses will watch you closely. When you are alert and comfortable, your family or friends may be allowed to be with you. After the nurses instruct your family or friends about your home care, you change back into your clothes and will be discharged.

Will I be in pain when I wake up from my anesthetic?

Plastic surgeons generally are excellent at placing local anesthesia in the affected surgical areas. Additionally, your anesthesia provider will be treating you with a combination of pain medicines in the operating room that will give you pain relief for the time you spend in the recovery room.

What can I eat after my surgery?

It is recommended that after you return home, you eat lightly the day of your surgery. Start off slowly with ample fluids such as water, light clear juices, electrolyte beverages (such as Gatorade), and foods such crackers and toast. Milk products, heavy, or greasy foods should be avoided. As you recover you may return to your regular diet.

Why can't I drive after surgery?

It is never a good idea to drive yourself home from surgery, as anesthesia can slow reflexes, slow your thought processes, and can even cause amnesia in the hours following surgery. So, while you may feel like yourself, your ability to drive and your judgment may be severely hampered. You must arrange for transportation and a caretaker prior to your surgery.

Medications utilized including prescription pain relievers, sedatives, muscle relaxants and many other medications, will slow your reflexes and affect your ability to drive safely. Your surgeon will advise you when it is safe to resume driving.

I'm afraid of general anesthesia. Could I die?

Most healthy people don't have any problems with general anesthesia. Although some people may have mild, temporary symptoms, general anesthesia itself is exceptionally safe, even for the sickest patients. In general, the risk of complications is more closely related to the type of procedure you're undergoing and your general physical health, rather than to the anesthesia itself.

The American Society of Anesthesiologists says a person is more likely to be struck by lightning than die from anesthesia-related complications. With state-of-the-art monitoring in an accredited surgical facility and anesthesia provided by an experienced board-certified anesthesiologist, safety and comfort have never been more reliable.

This chapter has covered most of the common questions patients ask about anesthesia-related issues. If you have more questions, you should consult your surgeon or anesthetic provider. A well-informed patient tends to be calmer around the time of surgery and oftentimes has fewer complications due to their understanding of the issues related to their care and recovery.

CHAPTER 18

What Patients Are Saying

"Dr. Ferrari is an amazing doctor. I would never go to a different doctor; you are the best! I will always recommend you and thank God there are surgeons like you that people can trust to do an incredible, safe and wonderful job!"

"Dr. Ferrari was extremely professional, the office was beautiful and all of the nurses made me feel very comfortable from my pre surgery appointments all the way to my 1 year later follow up. The practice has a very convenient location; they do all of their surgeries in house and never made you wait a long time like you do at the regular doctor's office. Dr. Ferrari did a wonderful job on my surgery and I have never regretted it. The downtime was what I was worried about. Turns out there was nothing to be worried about. I was sore the next day but back to work! I was driving 2 days later. The soreness lasted about 2.5 weeks and I was back working out like normal on week 5. I chose the "gummy bear" implant, which is silicone. He put them over the muscle."

"Dr. Ferrari and his staff are amazing. They are very friendly and make you feel comfortable every step of the way. They make sure to answer all of your questions and provide you with all the information you need to make the best decision for you. The surgery was easy and the recovery and results even better. I couldn't have picked a better team and wouldn't go anywhere else."

"Dr. Ferrari and his staff provided me with excellent care. Dr. Ferrari is an excellent surgeon and he is a very caring and compassionate doctor. His nurse Jenny is absolutely wonderful! She is so helpful through everything. I am so happy that I chose Dr. Ferrari to do my surgery. I am very happy with my results."

"Dr. Ferrari was the second doctor I visited for a breast augmentation consultation, and I knew right away that he was the right choice for me. He and his staff immediately put me at ease and made themselves available for questions and concerns in advance of my surgery. I was particularly impressed that Dr. Ferrari personally responded so quickly to the (many!) questions I emailed him in those couple of weeks. The day of surgery went smoothly, and I have been thrilled with my recovery and especially my results. I feel like I have the body I was always supposed to have! I can't say enough about Dr. Ferrari and his staff."

"Dr. Ferrari and his staff were terrific! They made me feel very comfortable and explained everything in great detail. My breast aug and lift turned out more beautiful than I imagined was even possible! I will definitely come back for my lipo and tummy tuck!"

"Dr. Ferrari is a very talented doctor. He is knowledgeable, patient and skillful. I'm glad I chose him. His staff is friendly and caring. He simply did an amazing job on my revision; he managed to shape the natural looking breasts I always wanted to have. I wish he had performed my very first augmentation so that I wouldn't need a second one."

"Dr. Ferrari and staff are very professional made me feel comfortable throughout the whole process and offered great advise. I am very pleased with my natural looking results. I would not go to a different doctor and recommend Dr. Ferrari to all my friends. Thanks Dr. Ferrari you are amazing!"

"Dr. Ferrari performed a breast lift, replacing my implants, and reduced the skin on my upper eyelids. He was the 4th Dr. that I interviewed. He was kind, courteous and extremely knowledgeable. He also spoke of a procedure for the lift that no other Dr. mentioned, reducing scarring and making it much more desirable for me. A year later, I don't know which I am happier about, my breasts or my eyes. I love them both!!! Thank you, Dr. Ferrari, and your wonderful staff. You all really are the BEST!"

"In my opinion, one of the best plastic surgeons in the country. I found Dr. Ferrari to be a very good listener that wanted to hear what I wanted for myself. He asked me a lot of questions and determined with Botox and an upper eye lift, I could achieve a younger look - and most important to me - a NATURAL look. I decided to go ahead and have Dr. Ferrari do the procedures. I would absolutely recommend Dr. Victor Ferrari without hesitation. He's a professional, skilled physician that listened to my needs and got me amazing results. I have recommended him to several co-workers and they have all been exceedingly pleased with his results. Thank you Dr. Ferrari and staff for your caring, expert work. I love that with the help of Dr. Ferrari I look 14 years younger than my age! Thank you, thank you!!"

"I have nothing but positive things to say about Dr. Ferrari and his staff. Dr. Ferrari is a consummate professional, who treated me with the utmost respect and care. I had a bad prior experience with another surgeon, so needless to say I had some major hesitancy in having my breast surgery revision. I can see why he is known as the best in what he does, because he is and it shows. I am so happy with my results; I am pleasantly surprised with how great I look and feel only 6 weeks after surgery. I would recommend him to anyone who is looking for a plastic surgeon."

"I had my surgery done five years ago but I would have to give Dr. Ferrari FIVE STARS in all categories. I had numerous consultations over a span of about 4 years before meeting and choosing Dr. Ferrari for my breast augmentation to correct severe asymmetry. When I visited the office for the first time, Dr. Ferrari took about 30 to 45 minutes to thoroughly discuss my issues. Through several more conversations, in person, by email & phone, he helped me formulate the best plan of action for my specific problem. He truly seemed to care, didn't ever rush me & did not treat me like just another number; unable to even acknowledge me in the hallway as the other doctors I had met with previously had. I live about an hour away from Charlotte, NC - where his office is located - but I looked forward each and every visit there. His staff at the time, were most courteous and helpful, never making me feel uncomfortable in the least. I had a wonderful experience from Premier Plastic Surgery with Dr. Victor Ferrari!"

About the Author

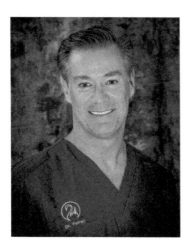

Dr. Victor S. Ferrari is the owner of and practices at Premier Plastic Surgery in Matthews, North Carolina, a suburb of Charlotte. He is a graduate of Davidson College, with honors. After completing four years of medical school at the University of North Carolina (Chapel Hill), Dr. Ferrari completed a full five-year general surgery residency at the University of Kansas and then three years of plastic surgery residency at one of the top programs in the country, the University of Miami. He then went on to a six-month craniofacial training program at Miami Children's Hospital. He not only served in the coveted position of Chief Resident in both specialties, but he also obtained board certification by the American Board of Surgery (1993-2004) and The American Board of Plastic Surgeons (1997 to present).

Dr. Ferrari was also elected to the American College of Surgeons that bestows the highest honors on those who are seen to be outstanding in their field. Five times he was awarded the "Physicians Recognition Award" by the American Medical Association. He has also been featured in many publications from the Consumers' Research Council, such as "Guide to America's Top Plastic Surgeons."

Dr. Ferrari has also been featured on numerous television and news shows including being the first plastic surgeon in the Charlotte area to be involved in a televised "Extreme Makeover" on FOX-TV. He performs most of his procedures in his own private nationally accredited in-office surgical facility or at Matthews Medical Center (formerly Presbyterian Hospital-Matthews).

For a consultation or more information about Dr. Victor Ferrari and Premier Plastic Surgery Center, visit http://www.Natural-LookingResults.com.

CPSIA information can be obtained
at www.ICGtesting.com
Printed in the USA
BVOW11s0958050517
483273BV00004B/5/P